About The Author

Dr E.A. Freeman is an Australian graduate of Sydney University. He also holds a Fellowship of the Royal College of Surgeons, Edinburgh. He and his wife and family spent seven years in Vanuatu in the South Pacific where Dr Freeman was a medical missionary.

He has been committed to those who are brain injured, and their relatives, since 1979. He was a co-investigator into the use of coma intervention as an adjunct to the management of the severely brain injured at a major Sydney teaching hospital. Currently, he is a director of the Australian Brain Foundation and a Medical Director of the Brain Injury Division of that organization. He now directs a Brain Injury Therapy Centre in Sydney.

1

To
Dorothy

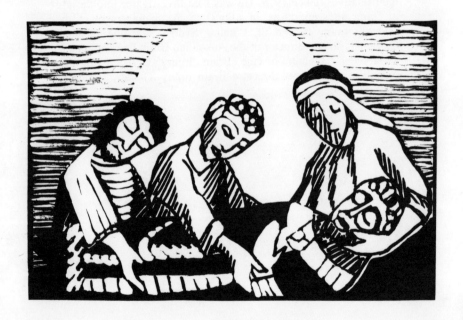

THE
CATASTROPHE
OF
COMA
a way back

E.A. Freeman
MB. BS. FRCS (Ed.)

David Bateman
Australia/New Zealand

First published in 1987 by
David Bateman Ltd.,
P.O. Box 257, Buderim,
Queensland 4556, Australia

National Library of Australia
Cataloguing-in-Publication data

Freeman, E.A.
    The Catastrophe of Coma: a way back

ISBN 0 949135 16 X

1. Coma — Patients — Rehabilitation.
I. Title.

616.8'49

Typeset by Lazerprintz, Auckland
Printed in Hong Kong by Colorcraft

CONTENTS

What you need when you are lost — A Map — A Diary — A Guide — Relatives and Friends — A Roster — Hope — You and the Patient — Action sheet.

BRAIN INJURY — WHAT IS IT?

Head Injury or Brain Injury? — Types of Head Injury — Why the Brain Gets Injured — Types of Brain Injury — The Initial Damage — The Secondary Damage — The Intracranial Pressure — Extradural Haemorrhage — Subdural Haemorrhage — Intracerebral Haemorrhage.

MEASURING THE PATIENT'S CONDITION AND WHAT IT MEANS

Coma — The Glasgow Coma Scale — Motor Response — Eye-opening — Pupil Size — Vocal Response — Age — Other Important Factors — Coming Out of Coma.

WHAT HAPPENS IN INTENSIVE CARE?

The Tubes Attached to the Patient — The Breathing Tube — The Feeding Tube — The Intravenous Lines — The Intracranial Monitor — The Catheter — The Tubes in the Chest — Drugs.

THE THINGS THAT CAN'T BE CHANGED AND
THE THINGS THAT CAN BE CHANGED

Fixed Factors — The Primary Brain Injury — The Age of the Patient — Non-Fixed Factors — The Micro-environment — The Macro-environment — The Changing Problem — How our Brain Works — The Cybernetic Loop — Sensory Deprivation.

WHAT TO DO IN THE UNCONSCIOUS AND RESPONSIVE
PATIENT — MOTOR OUTPUT

The Importance of Movement — The Regaining of Motor Function — The Patient with No Movement or with Reflex Movement — The Patient Out of Coma with No Movement or Reflex Movement — The Patient Out of Coma with Spontaneous Movement or Controlled Movement — The Importance of the Central Axis — The Position of the Head — Moving the Central Axis — The Legs — Protecting the Central Axis — The Arms — Hand Function — The Grasp Reflex — The Grasp Release — The Prehensile Grasp — The Pincer Grasp — Speech — Feeding

SECTION F   PROLONGED COMA   219

CHAPTER 23   220

PROLONGED COMA — THE PERSISTENT VEGETATIVE STATE
THE LOCKED-IN STATE

Definition of Persistent Vegetative State — The Incidence of PVS — Is it Possible to Identify PVS Accurately? — The Effect of the Diagnosis of PVS on the Patient, Relatives, Profession — How the System Deals with the PVS Patient — What Should be the Approach — The Diagnosis — The Management — The Trial of Arousal — The Definition of the Locked-In State — The Approaches to the Patient in the Locked-In State.

SECTION G   OTHER IMPORTANT INFORMATION   232

CHAPTER 24   233

ASPECTS OF THE TRADITIONAL MANAGEMENT AND THE
OUTCOME OF SEVERE BRAIN INJURY

The Importance of Early Resuscitation — Survival and General Outcome — Function and Outcome.

CHAPTER 25   239

HOW DOES THE PATIENT FEEL?

The Approach to the Relative — The Recollections of the Patient — The Inadvertent Remarks — The Failure to Help — The Factors of Importance.

HOW DO THE RELATIVES COPE?

Reality — The Reality of the Patient — Reality for You — Mental Resources — Self-talk — Other People's Talk — Visualisation — Meditation — Forgiveness — The Importance of the NOW — Physical Wellbeing — Social Wellbeing — Spiritual Growth — Faith — Hope — Love — Failure — Conclusion.

WHAT MAY BEAT YOU IN THE SYSTEM AND HOW TO DEAL WITH IT

The Background to the Medical System — The Severely Brain-injured and the System — Time — Place — People — Dealing with the Physician — Medical Ethics and Informed Consent — Other Organisations.

CONCLUSION

The Caring Professions and the Patient — The Caring Professions and the Relatives — To the Relatives and Friends — The Reason for Writing — The Moral Problems.

FOREWORD

This book comes at a time when the whole field of medicine is in a state of turmoil. The reasons are many. The amazing growth of scientific and technological skill in the healing profession has taken place against the backdrop of an equal growth in the expectations and demands of modern man as regards health. Popular publications carry news of every new advance, while the general concept grows that there must be a panacea for every ill, a cure for every disease, and we want that answer NOW. Meanwhile the field which was once dominated by caring and charitable concern has increasingly yielded to drive towards commercial and industrial dominants, profits, mass production and mechanisation.

Going hand in hand with this general feeling about the advance of science, however, there is a paradox. Science too poses the greatest threats to man's sense of security and his hopes for the future. Not only atomic power but the growing assaults on the environment and the unknowns of counter-reactions to new medical preparations are just part of this fear. Seemingly impregnable viruses arise which bring abrupt and fundamental changes to the modern life-style.

Genetic engineering and man's capacity to interfere with laws of cause and effect as old as evolution raise miasmic spectres at least in the shadowy background of our minds.

Nevertheless, across the world today there is a growing realisation that the individual's health, healing from disease and wounds of mind and body and the capacity to cope with one's environment, all have to do with a holistic or fully rounded view of the human person. Not only the needs of the physical body but realising and engaging the power and input of the mind and 'spirit' of a person are vital to any healing concept. The human mind is addressed in various ways, of which intellect, emotions and willpower are major factors. Researchers in all the human sciences — such as education and psychology all point towards the vital importance of factors such as love, hope, purpose, understanding, and faith in integrating the human individual in his or her fight against the impairment of the person, at even the most patently physical level.

A leading Japanese medical researcher, Kintaro Shigozukyi, said recently:

> "Scientific thinking, which has made such a basic impact upon the wider human thoughts of the world and human nature, and is now taking up life itself as the central issue, will expand its area of interest and will view the object in totality, rather than just a part . . . Thus the scientific concept and its methodology will become basically different in its approach to its objects."

Dr. Freeman has been fighting for this holistic approach to severe brain injury for almost a decade. In doing so he has encountered an astonishing amount of opposition. At the time this book goes to print however, the worst of that battle seems to be over. A leading Melbourne neuro-surgeon, John Woodward, who died recently at a tragically early age, has followed and encouraged Freeman's work for some years. As a Director of the Australian Brain Foundation he was asked to do so by the Board of Directors of that body. Just before he died in 1987, Mr. Woodward wrote to me as Chairman of the Division of the Brain Foundation facilitating Freeman's work:

". . . my part in the Division's development these past few years has been among the really exciting things, and it pleased me no end to see your little organisation reaching a point at which at last it becomes 'unstoppable'. Sincere good luck to everyone concerned, and thank you for having me as a colleague in what I recognize to be a very important venture."

As I write these few words I have just come from viewing a video presentation from the United States where a great chain of institutions is being developed to begin treating the tens of thousands of young persons with severe brain injuries who have been languishing in nursing homes and terminal care institutions because medicine had no effective way to treat them. Today, prominent in their new approach, are the cardinal points outlined in this book: — early intervention, as soon as possible after the patient's life has been secured following the accident; the vital role of the nearest relatives; the aggressive use of sensory and physical stimulation and, above all, the atmosphere of loving care and encouragement.

Prof. Gerald Jampolsky M.D. writes: "It is clear to most physicians that attitude can affect organic illness. They know that the will to live or die can change the course of an illness. They know this, though such an attitude cannot be put under a microscope, measured, weighed or replicated. The truths of the mind defy the usual standards of science."

On my desk is a translation of an address given in Korea recently by Dr. Shigozuyki as the Secretary General of the Japanese Christian Medical Fellowship in his keynote address to a world congress in 1986, in which he says, *inter alia*:

"The remarkable progress in scientific knowledge and technological skill in recent years are helping us to discover many new dimensions of the surrounding environment and of human nature which were not properly known to us before. It is now necessary to make some alterations or new additions to the concepts and methodology which were taken for granted as scientific common sense for many years. These days we are so overwhelmed by the scientific knowledge and technology that we are almost too intimidated to face up to the new experiences, or to speak about them in public, when they don't seem to fit in with the so-called scientific common-sense of our time. We tend to ignore or even despise such experiences and people who take them so seriously, simply because they cannot be explained by our own limited experiences or by the scientific knowledge which we understand . . . We are now gradually searching for new and deeper dimensions of human nature. Needless to say, this does not mean bringing any unscientific elements into science itself, nor limiting the scientific enquiry of human experiences. On the contrary, we expect to see the horizon of the concept and method of enquiry being expanded and deepened to accommodate the new discoveries and experiences."

When you read this book, you will possibly feel as I do, that it is a temporary measure only. This for two reasons:

A. There is still a long way to go before long-held and entrenched prejudices are overcome in many sectors of the healing professions. It would be nice to be able to wait until the great majority were convinced and were applying such measures in areas where there is little hope otherwise.

That is not possible, especially for those of us who have had the tragedy of severe brain injury hurtle into our lives and that of our family. Such people want help NOW, and our research so far indicates that the longer the kind of help outlined in this book is delayed the more difficult the healing process and the more dismal the prospect for recovery.

B. By the same token, it can only be a matter of time, hopefully a short time, before the mounting volume of evidence of a wholly new prospect for the brain-injured leads to widespread acceptance by the medical profession as a whole.

Meanwhile this book will enable loved-ones to receive from those we find best fitted to give it, the kind of encouragement and stimulation they desperately need when they are rendered so suddenly less able to deal with themselves and their environment than even a new born babe.

Have faith, hope, and love. Without them no therapy can heal the person. They are the very life-blood of human existence. The greatest of them all is love — and the most powerful.

11th April, 1987.

Malcolm G. Mackay, A.M., B.A., B.D., PhD.
Chairman,
Brain Injury Division,
Australian Brain Foundation,
Canberra.

ACKNOWLEDGEMENTS

Many people have contributed to the information provided in this book and to them, I give my warmest thanks and my gratitude.

The book was written in response to requests from relatives of the brain-injured who sought some written guidance to help their loved one come out of coma and regain normal living.

It was these relatives who ventured into the unknown areas of coma with the original Coma Arousal Team at The Westmead Hospital in Sydney, Australia and from them I learnt the value of the relatives in providing that "loving cocoon" for the fragile patient arousing from coma.

They were my guide — my eyes, my ears, my hands, my thoughts as I laboured to frame up, in some acceptable way, the knowledge which they alone could obtain. Frequently, I stood in wonder and awe as they demonstrated what they could obtain from the patient where I had failed. I sat at their feet and learnt. I also marvelled and was humbled by their strength of purpose. Not all of them succeeded in what they were attempting and I shared their sorrow. With those who did succeed, I shared their joy.

The work entailed in developing the methods in this book could not have eventuated without the Coma Arousal Nurses; Mrs Beverly Burrell, who bore the full brunt in the early stages, along with Mrs Yvonne Ayrey, Mrs Liz Reynolds, Mr Gary Burnes, Mrs Marlene Prince, Mrs Robyn Sedger, Mr Paul Healey, Mrs Maureen Lewsey and Ms Sandra Lever. Mr John Ayrey has contributed his thoughts as a patient and has contributed to the development of the questionnaire along with Ms Grace Sorbello and Mr John Walsh. To these people, I am very grateful.

The social workers, Mrs Anne MacLeay and Ms Liz Davies also contributed their skills in regard to many of the patients and fully supported the relatives.

Mr Peter Lipscombe, in a very gentle and sensitive way has videoed many of the patients — a tremendous help to our learning.

Perhaps this whole project may not have eventuated without the support of World Vision of Australia. It was Mr Harold Henderson, the Executive Director of that organisation, who provided the "seeding" funds at a critical time of great difficulty.

The Directors of the Brain Injury Division of the Australian Brain Foundation, especially the chairman, Dr Malcolm Mackay and Mrs Ruth Mackay have been supportive and encouraging throughout the preparation of this manuscript, providing many of the ideas expressed here and have sought constantly to ensure the ease of comprehension. Dr John Woodward of Melbourne guided me over many difficulties during the learning process of this book.

Mr Ian Hunt, the vice chairman, has consistently demanded that it be produced.

Mr Kevin Beckton and Mr John Green of the The New South Wales Government Insurance Office along with the chairman, Mr Bob Somervaille and the managing director, Mr Bill Jocelyn recognised the enormous potential of early intervention in the brain-injured patient. Not only did they see this as a financial responsibility but they have been deeply committed from the humane viewpoint.

The Rev. Marilyn Stacey has been of great assistance in perusing the manuscript and has helped to clarify some of the thinking expressed in the book.

The Rev. Alan Smart has provided sections of his sermons and has constantly initiated thought provoking ideas.

My thanks go also to Mrs Mary Maxwell who has maintained a harmonious state through all the drafts.

To Dr Edward Le Winn from the Institute for the Achievement of Human Potential, Philadelphia, I owe a large debt. When I visited him in 1979 and watched him working, I realised that a continuing negative approach to the brain-injured was not logical and could not be supported.

Mr Ian Hunter of The Australian Centre for Brain Injured Children has shared his knowledge with me willingly and I am indebted to him.

My publishers, David Bateman, have supported and guided the development of this book from its early stages. I am very grateful to Australian Director, Michael White, whose son was brain injured in 1984, and to David and Janet Bateman in New Zealand for all their help and advice.

The members of my family have been of enormous help. My wife Dorothy has drawn the frontispiece and Thomas the illustrations throughout the book. Dorothy has only once queried my working in this emotionally demanding field. Paraphrasing the words of G.K.Chesterton she has "Stuck to me through thick and thin; the thickness of my head and the thinness of my excuses." To my children, Matthew (1957-1980), Thomas, Susan, James, Jocelyn and Ross, I give my loving thanks for their support.

Sydney
May 20th, 1987.

E.A. Freeman

INTRODUCTION

YOU AND YOUR PART

Not a day passes over the earth,
but men and women of no note
do great deeds,
speak great words,
and suffer noble sorrows.

Charles Reade

YOU AND YOUR PART

This is a personal book. You have a personal problem. You need to know how to deal with it.

By the time this book is in your hands the catastrophe of what has happened to your son or daughter or husband or wife or brother or sister or father or mother or friend will have hit you.

The common statement that I have heard among relatives and friends of those who are severely brain injured is: "This is the worst thing that has ever happened to our family." That thought is the starting-point of reality for you and for the patient.

Let's start with you, since the patient is undoubtedly receiving the very best of medical and nursing care already in the Intensive Care Ward of the hospital.

You

It is an old and true saying that "the way forward is the way through". I often tell relatives of the brain-injured that they will need patience, courage and endurance. Words are always easy to say, it is the doing that is difficult. The story of humanity is full of the stories of people who have displayed these qualities.

Let me say that, in dealing with relatives of the brain-injured, it has been rare for anyone not to display that patience, courage and endurance. There are always times, of course, when we sink low in thoughts and feelings if we have a great problem. We have to accept these times, but realize that they do not last.

You may think that the people with whom I have dealt have been a selected group, abnormally strong mentally and physically, but this has not been so. They have been people of all ages and from all walks of life and they have all shown the same strength. Their financial background has ranged from wealthy to poor, but they have all shown great strength and courage.

Human endurance in time of great stress is a quality that I view with a great deal of humility and thankfulness. You may doubt that you have this inner strength. I can assure you that it is present, but it usually needs to be directed.

How do you feel now? The answer is, probably, terrible. I suppose that it is very much like the feeling of being lost, and that can be a terrible feeling. In a way you are lost, lost in a system that is totally foreign to you and over which you have no control.

Despair comes upon us so easily and begins to eat away at our very being. Despair is a bad feeling, for it takes away hope, and without hope there can be no tomorrow.

As one American writer put it in regard to brain injury: "It is impossible to remain aloof when faced with a family torn by fright and anger, handicapped by guilt and denial and seemingly abandoned by a system that doesn't care enough."

These words will probably apply to you. You will be torn with fright and anger:

frightened, because you don't know what's going on; angry, because you appear to have no power in the decisions which are being made; handicapped, because there is always something that you should have done better with the person you love before the accident took place, and you will feel guilty about this and handicapped by the denial of the reality of what has occurred — "Why-did-this-happen?" syndrome.

So you are lost in a system which, at first, seems to be beyond comprehension and understanding.

What you need when you are lost

1. A Map

When you are lost, what you need desperately is a map, and, if possible, someone to give you guidance until you are safe.

When you look at a map, the first thing you do is to find out where you are. This is the first step to reality. You do this by looking for places with which you are familiar, and which you can use to point you in the right direction.

If you are on a journey, then you expect to use the map more than just once. You know that you will be referring to it repeatedly, to ensure that you are on the right path.

You will also use a map to plan your way ahead, and then to see how far you have come and how much farther there is to go. Any journey takes time, and you are on one of the most important journeys of your life, and much is at stake.

This book aims to provide you with a map and to indicate in which direction you should go. It is rough in places, because much of the ground you will cover is in uncharted areas, and the journey which you make will be different from that made by any other person.

2. A Diary

Start your diary today. In it you record:

1. The facts that you have been told about the patient.
2. The things that you have seen about the patient.
3. How you feel about what you have been told.
4. How you feel about the patient.
5. Other facts that are important to you (e.g., how the rest of the family is coping).

You don't need a fancy book for this. An exercise book will do.

Ask all relatives and friends who see the patient to write their observations in this book. Ask them to do it each time they visit. This book becomes most important as your record of what has happened. It should be done each day. It provides you with written information, which you need, since so much will occur each day that you will not be able to remember it. Yet you need to remember everything.

Your diary will help you when you become despondent, and worried that there is no improvement, and you will be able to look back to a week or a month before and see how far the patient has come. The diary will also allow you to get your thoughts in order at the end of each day, and will encourage you to be realistic. It will present the facts on paper and release you mentally from mulling them over again and again.

When you have recorded the observations, you should attempt to convince yourself that the day's work is done in this regard, and you should get on and do something completely different. This is difficult to do, but if you have other family to attend to, then you should give them time. You should also try to maintain contact with your friends. When the diary is written, that is the time to cut off from the problems of the day.

3. A Guide

A book *The Wounded Healer* by Father Henri Nouwen, Image Books 1979, tells you the value of talking to someone who has suffered similarly. It is wise to seek out someone who has experienced the same situation and suffered the same trauma. That person can be your guide.

Don't forget that you are different from your helper and guide. The brain injured person you love is also different in personality and in the type and extent of the brain injury from anyone else, so take the positives that your helper can give and shy away from any negatives they may express.

There are others who will also be of considerable help; medical, nursing, social-work people and other hospital staff.

4. Relatives and Friends

You will have to make an effort with your relatives and friends, because they will not know how to deal with you in this situation. They may tend to withdraw, not because they have ceased to like you, but because they do not wish to intrude. Or they may be so concerned to know what is happening that they will be on the telephone to you even at the most inappropriate times.

What you don't want is to be barraged by the phone every time you are home, to have to repeat the story over and over to many people at the end of the day, or even during the day. It is better to seek help from a few relatives and friends and ask them to relay the messages on the patient's state to those involved. Some people will be upset by not being able to talk to you directly, but do not be worried by this. You cannot afford to be inundated with telephone calls.

5. A Roster

Because so much of the future of the patient and your family will eventually depend on how you handle this catastrophe, you must identify your family resources and allocate them correctly and productively.

In the initial few days, during the life threatened stage, it is likely that all the family will want to gather at the hospital and support each other and the patient, and this is necessary and valuable. When it becomes apparent that the patient is very likely to survive, you must conserve your resources so that you will be able to provide the support for the patient over the weeks and months ahead. If you all stay at the bedside, you will become tired, angry, irritable and frustrated, and you will come into conflict with each other and wear each other out. This would be disastrous for the patient and for your own family group.

To avoid this one of the family should draft a roster which will both provide adequate bedside coverage for the patient and allow all members time away from the hospital to work or attend to the rest of the living of the family.

You can also harness the community in this way. If you are a small family, then bring in school friends, church friends, club friends, work friends. In one very rewarding instance, the small but loving family of a young soldier sought and received excellent support from the armed forces.

This roster should be done on a weekly basis, planned to provide the necessary input to the patient but flexible enough to allow change. It should be done by the Thursday for the following week, so that all are aware of their commitment and any necessary alterations can be made.

It is preferable that no one stays for more than four hours at the bedside; otherwise the psychological burden can be too heavy, though this will depend upon the condition of the patient and the feelings of the person involved.

6. Hope

There are other factors of great importance. The three which spring to mind immediately are faith, hope and love.

We know that love is there, otherwise you would not be involved. It is the mainspring for everything else. Faith is very personal. It is dealt with in a later chapter. Hope is what I wish to talk about now. We all need hope. Hope gives us a vision for the future, and we need that vision.

You will find that many people will not wish to give you hope, because they will honestly believe that there is no hope, or that there is very little. You must listen to them and weigh up what they say, but remember they are usually talking from a statistical point of view and you are dealing from a personal point of view. While they have good reason for presenting the honest picture to you, they are talking in terms of numbers of people, not in terms of your patient, your loved one. Do not argue with them, because they cannot change what they are telling you. It is what they honestly believe. They are not trying to deceive you.

There are reasons why you should continue to hope, and I shall present them as simply as I can.

The *first* is that you can't help it. It is a natural response, and you cannot wipe it away, no matter how much you try. It is like someone telling you to stop breathing. You just can't help having some hope, no matter how small.

The *second* is that this problem will govern the whole of your outlook and attitude to your life, to the life of your family and to the life of the patient. You know that you can't walk away and forget about the problem. It confronts your every waking moment. It dominates your life.

The *third* reason is that perhaps, in some indefinable way, you transmit to the patient your own feelings. It may be that the loving bond between you and the injured person, which has been there since birth or for decades, allows some communication in an as-yet-unknown manner between you. It is almost as if vibes, which can't be seen or measured, connect the patient and relatives. The existence of these has not been validated, but to most people they are real and functioning. In fact, a majority of relatives interviewed would believe that patient has some awareness of them, even when no one else in the medical or nursing team shares their belief.

One researcher has commented on this in dealing with patients who were in prolonged coma when he says, "There always remains the lingering doubt that the patient might in fact have some mental activity, which we have simply failed to detect; this doubt is often kindled by claims from those caring for the vegetative wreck on a full-time basis that the patient actually makes himself understood in an uncommon or even eerie way." (Bricolo A, Turazzi S, Feriotti G. Prolonged Post traumatic Unconsciousness *J. Neurosurgery*, 52; 625-634 1980)

Your attitude may, therefore, have a significant bearing on the rate and extent of recovery of the patient. This is only theoretical, but it should be regarded as possible, until either proven or disproven. It is better to err on the side of belief than to discount this possibility.

The *fourth* reason is that medicine is not an absolute science. It does not know all. The area of brain injury is undergoing intense scrutiny all over the world, and more knowledge is constantly being gained.

In some parts of the globe there is a movement away from the fatalistic approach of "there is nothing to be done" to a more positive attitude to brain injury.

You and the Patient

The patient will go through four major stages of care. We shall be looking at the first stage only in this chapter. This is the stage of acute care.

Most severely brain-injured patients go under the care of a neurosurgeon (see Chapter 4). The standard of care is very good. Usually the patient has first been seen and assessed in the Emergency Ward of the hospital and then sent to the the the Operating Theatre, if that is necessary, and/or to the Intensive Care Unit. The care in all these areas is of the very highest medical and nursing standard.

The Intensive Care Unit will be a shock, The sight of so many very sick people gathered together, connected up to many different machines that breathe for them, maintain their blood pressure, etc., can be shattering. It can be shattering for those who work there, and even members of the medical and nursing profession who are familiar with all the equipment and monitors can be very emotionally upset when they see a person whom they love in such a place.

For those who are totally unfamiliar with the scene, apart from watching TV medical shows, the effect can be devastating. Many feel very uneasy and faint. This is nothing to be embarrassed about. It can happen to anyone. It is your "hot brain" dominating you(see Chapter 5). What you need now is information to get your cold brain going. I'll be explaining these terms in the next chapter.

You should ask to see the person who is looking after your patient. It is unlikely that the neurosurgeon will be there to talk to you, but you should seek the most senior person in the Intensive Care Unit. They are all very busy, but they will know how distraught you are and will make time for you. You could have to wait, for there may be duties relating to other patients, which must take priority over a discussion with you.

In this time it is useful to make up a check list of what you wish to know. If you have a chance to read any literature on brain injury, then do so, so you will have some understanding of what the doctor is describing.

Basically what you are going to ask is:

1. How extensive is the damage?
2. How severe is the damage?
3. Is his /her life still threatened?
4. How long will he/she be in coma?
5. What is the likely outcome of the injury? In other words, what will he/she be like in six months, or a year, or two years?

You will, unfortunately, not get many answers to these questions, for the plain fact is that the doctors or staff will not know. They may be able to give you an idea of the severity of the brain injury, but may not be sure of the extent. The doctor will be able to tell you if the life of the patient is still threatened, but will not be able to predict with any accuracy how long the patient will be in coma.

The doctor will not be able to tell you what the prognosis is for the future. It is not a matter of evading telling you the truth, but of genuinely not knowing. This may come as a shock, as you have probably been led to believe that the medical profession knows all about the injured body. Unfortunately, this is not so. Do not argue with the doctor, even if you disagree. You are being told what has been learnt from medical training and experience.

You can do only three things. WAIT and PRAY and ACT.

It is very likely that if you are present soon after the accident, the patient is in a life-threatened state, and this time of waiting becomes interminable. It seems to go on for ever. You know that your patient is in the very best of medical and nursing hands, and that is all the information that you really now have.

Whether you wish to wait at the bedside, or in the room outside the Intensive Care Unit, is up to you. Often it is better to limit yourself in this early stage to brief visits to the unit. To stay in there for too long can be very depressing.

When you go into the waiting-room in a big hospital, you will possibly meet someone in a similar position. The injury to the person whom they love will probably be different from the injury to the person whom you love, but they will have been through some of the same emotional trauma. It can do you a lot of good to talk to someone else. This person probably knows what facilities the hospital has: where the cafe is, the coffee rooms, the toilets, etc.

The social worker will probably make contact with you at this time to give you help in sorting out any problems which you and your family may have both inside and outside the hospital.

The hospital may have rooms for relatives of the very sick, and you may be able to obtain accommodation. It is worthwhile asking the social worker about this. They may not be able to provide it immediately, but will try to ensure that your name is placed on the list for it.

If you can, you should get out and go for a walk at least every morning and afternoon for a half hour or so. This will help you relax.

As the days go by, the chances of survival improve. You may also feel that there is some indication that the patient is waking up. You may be the only one who thinks so, your opinion may not be shared by the medical and nursing staff, but do not be put off by this. Often you will be told that certain things you observe happening are merely coincidence. They may be, but if you keep seeing movements, or facial expression, then note them all down in your diary. If you can have a witness to these happenings, that is better. If you can't, then still look for them.

One thing which worries many people is that, when they put their hand into the hand of the patient, they feel a movement. This is very likely to be a reflex, the grasp reflex, and should not be taken as a sign that the patient is awake. It is purely a reflex, but a reflex is better than nothing.

Take note of all things — of any movement — and record it in your diary.

ACTION SHEET

1. HOLD ON TO HOPE.

2. START YOUR DIARY.

3. ORGANISE YOUR TELEPHONE.

4. ORGANISE YOUR ROSTER.

5. START TO REORGANISE YOUR LIFE.

6. KEEP YOURSELF FIT.

7. SEEK A FORMAL MEETING WITH THE DOCTOR IN CHARGE.

8. SCAN CHAPTER 1 AND CHAPTER 2.

9. AT THE MEETING WITH THE DOCTOR ASK HIM OR HER TO

    1. MARK THE TYPE OF INJURY IN YOUR BOOK.

    2. TELL YOU OF OTHER INJURIES.

        WRITE THEM DOWN HERE;

        1.

        2.

        3.

    3. INDICATE THE GENERAL CONDITION OF THE PATIENT.

    4. LIST THE PATIENT ON THE GLASGOW COMA SCALE.

SECTION A

THE PATIENT AND BRAIN INJURY

CHAPTER 1

BRAIN INJURY — WHAT IS IT?

This chapter will explain what has happened to the person whom you love, and what is being done to help that person.

Your doctor at the hospital should give you a detailed account of what has happened. The aim here is to give you a general understanding of what has occurred. It will also help you to know what questions to ask.

Ask your doctor if there is anything that you do not understand. S/He will be pleased to explain.

Head Injury or Brain Injury?

These are two sets of KEY WORDS:

    HEAD INJURY
    BRAIN INJURY

You will often hear that someone has a head injury, and this is understood to mean brain injury. There is a difference, however.

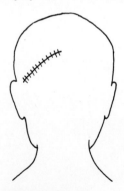

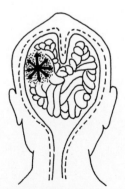

HEAD INJURY
May not affect
the brain.

BRAIN INJURY
Always affects
the brain.

Fig. 1.1

Head injury can mean brain injury, but it can also mean injury to the face, scalp, ears, skull, etc., with only minor injury to the brain, or with none at all. A person can have a laceration (cut) to the face, or a contusion (bruising) to the scalp, which is called a head injury, but which is unlikely to cause any severe brain injury.

Some patients who have few marks on their head may have a serious brain injury. They may look perfectly all right on the outside of the head, but have a very serious problem inside the skull.

Head injuries without brain injury are not likely to cause death or serious disability; they may cause problems of appearance, but the patient is unlikely to die.

Brain injury is different. Brain injury can cause very severe illness and in some cases can lead to death.

Types of Head Injury

These are the KEY WORDS:

CLOSED HEAD INJURY
OPEN HEAD INJURY

A head injury is called a *closed head injury* if there is no break through the skull, and this is similar to a stroke or cerebrovascular accident. If there is a break in the skull, it is called a *penetrating head injury*, or *open head injury*. A major problem with the open type head injury is that infection may track from the outside of the skull into the brain, causing brain abscesses, or meningitis. Antibiotics are usually given to these patients.

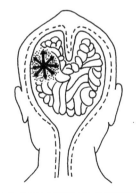

CLOSED HEAD INJURY
Brain not open to air.

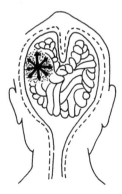

OPEN HEAD INJURY
Brain open to air.

Fig. 1.2

The Brain

These are the KEY WORDS:

MENINGES
(Coverings of the brain)

                    1 Dura mater
                    2 Pia mater
                    3 Arachnoid mater

INTRACEREBRAL   Inside the brain
THE BRAINSTEM   The part of the brain that
                    connects to the spinal cord.

The brain is soft, like a very firm jelly, and it sits inside the skull, which is the bony box protecting it. The brain doesn't just flop around inside the skull; it is held in place by three different coverings called the meninges.

The outermost and thickest of these linings is called the dura mater (pronounced *dew-ra mar-tar*). It is like a piece of canvas that holds the brain in place in the midline, so it won't shift too much from side to side. One part of the brain also sits on this canvas-like substance, as if it were a hammock (see Fig 1.3). The other two linings (the pia mater and the arachnoid mater) aren't very thick, but they have a layer of fluid between them called the cerebrospinal fluid (C.S.F.), which allows the brain to float like a boat on water.

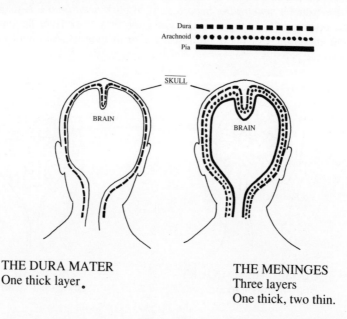

THE DURA MATER
One thick layer.

THE MENINGES
Three layers
One thick, two thin.

Fig. 1.3

Any sudden jolts or knocks to the brain are reduced, because the shock-wave is taken up by this cerebrospinal fluid.

The brainstem is a very important part of the brain in terms of evolution. It is a very old part of the brain and connects it with the spinal cord. Therefore the nerves that join the body and brain go through the brainstem to the brain. It also contains the parts of the brain which control our breathing, swallowing, temperature and blood pressure.

The brain needs a very good supply of blood. Almost 20 per cent of the blood pumped from the heart goes to the brain. Some of the blood vessels in the skull run up between the skull and the thick lining, the dura mater; others run through the space in which the C.S.F. is, the so-called subarachnoid space (pronounced *sub-arak-noid* space) and through this to the brain surface and deep into the brain.

Why the brain gets injured

When the head is hit, or strikes an object, the scalp can be damaged, the skull can be bruised or fractured (broken), and the force sent on to the brain. If the force of impact is strong, the shock-absorber effect of the fluid will not work effectively. The brain coverings will not protect the brain sufficiently, and the brain will hit against the inside of the skull and be damaged. The skull does not need to be broken for this type of damage to occur.

Sometimes the brain is actually torn by the brain coverings, as they attempt to hold the brain in place, and at other times the blood vessels are broken and torn. In some cases the skull is fractured (broken), and the broken bone of the skull is pushed into the brain.

At times the *brainstem* can be injured with very little damage to the rest of the brain. The brainstem contains within it the arousal mechanism of the brain, a very important structure called the Reticular Activating System. It is considered to be the area on which anaesthetics work to produce the unconscious state for operations to be performed. When it is damaged by brain injury, as it frequently is, by being either stretched, or twisted or compressed, the patient loses consciousness. Many hold the opinion that it is only when the Activating System regains function, that coma ceases and consciousness returns.

Types of brain injury

The KEY WORDS in types of brain injury are as follows:

THE INITIAL DAMAGE	at time of injury.
THE SECONDARY DAMAGE	at some period after the accident.
FOCAL BRAIN INJURY	injury which is focused on one part of the brain.
DIFFUSE BRAIN INJURY	widespread damage to the brain.
BRAINSTEM INJURY	injury to the brainstem.
INTRACRANIAL PRESSURE	pressure inside the skull.
INTRACRANIAL HAEMORRHAGE	bleeding inside the skull.

HAEMATOMA	collection of blood (blood clot).
INTRACRANIAL HAEMATOMA	collection of blood (clot) inside the skull.
CEREBRAL OEDEMA	swelling of the brain.

The effects of the damage

There are two main effects of brain injury. They are due to:

- the initial damage
- the secondary damage

The Initial Damage

The initial damage occurs when the brain cells are injured, and in some cases die, *at the time of the impact.* This damage is caused by direct injury to the brain when the bony skull hits it, or an object penetrates through the skull into the brain, or in some cases by a reduction of blood flow, or lack of oxygen to areas of the brain,

The injury may be called *diffuse brain injury* if it is widespread, or *localized brain injury* or *focal brain injury* if it is in one part of the brain or several separate sections of the brain. That is, *diffuse brain injury* means that the injury to the brain is widespread and involves many different areas of the brain. The opposite of diffuse brain injury is localized brain injury, where only a relatively small part of the brain is injured. Both types can occur together.

The Secondary Damage

The second type of damage to the brain occurs after the accident. Not all brain-injured patients have evidence of secondary damage. The extent of this type of damage can vary from very mild to very severe. Some people call it the "second accident".

(N.B. NOT ALL PATIENTS HAVE THIS "SECOND ACCIDENT")

When the brain is injured, it may swell up. This causes the pressure inside the skull to rise. We have said that the brain is soft, and sits inside a hard bony box, which is almost totally enclosed. When the pressure starts to rise inside the skull, it starts to squeeze on the brain, often forcing it down towards the top part of the spinal cord. This is known as *coning* (see Fig. 1.4).

When this happens, the brainstem, which is the part of the brain which controls our temperature and heart rate, and keeps us awake and breathing, finds it difficult to continue working. If the pressure continues to increase, and the brain is pushed farther down towards the spinal cord death can result, because these vital centres of control are put out of action as the blood supply is cut off.

The pressure inside the skull pushes the brain down towards the spinal cord.

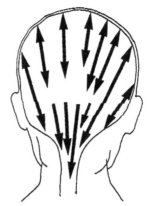

Fig. 1.4. CONING

It sometimes happens that a person can be hit on the head and get up, walk about and talk, and then become unconscious, owing to the effects of this "second accident". It is as if the first accident was not very severe, but has started off the process that leads to a rise in pressure inside the skull, which starts the squeeze on the brain. The period of time that the person is awake between the accident, and the time he becomes unconscious, is called the *lucid interval*.

It is possible for all the processes of brain injury to occur closely together. There can be brain-cell death owing to the effect of the first accident, followed by bleeding inside the skull and swelling of the brain owing to the "second accident".

Secondary damage can also be caused by problems in other parts of the body. If the lungs or blood circulation have been injured, the brain may be unable to obtain enough oxygen. Sometimes also there can be bleeding into the brain a week or so after the first accident. This is known as *delayed* or *secondary* haemorrhage.

The Intracranial Pressure

The KEY WORDS here are:

EXTRADURAL	outside the dura mater and, therefore, between the dura mater and the skull.
SUBDURAL	underneath the dura mater.
SUBARACHNOID	under the arachnoid mater.
INTRACEREBRAL	inside the substance of the brain.

The cerebrospinal fluid inside the skull has a positive pressure called the *intracranial pressure*. While most people are familiar with blood pressure measurements being taken with the use of a mercury blood pressure instrument, pressure of the c.s.f. in the brain is much less than blood pressure and is measured with an instrument using water as its measuring fluid. The pressure of the c.s.f. will normally not raise a column of water in an instrument more than 18-20 cms. A rise

31

in intracranial pressure in those who are brain injured is usually caused either by:

- the brain swelling, known as cerebral oedema (*cerebral* meaning brain, and *oedema* meaning swelling). It really means that there is too much fluid being kept in the brain, and the brain is incapable of getting rid of it.

    or

- bleeding inside the skull, called *intracranial haemorrhage*.

In the latter, if the bleeding continues, it can lead to a collection of blood called a haematoma, which may form a clot in or on the outside of the brain. The bleeding may be mainly from arteries or from veins, or the small blood vessels called capillaries which connect the two. Because blood in the arteries is at a high pressure, the pressure inside the skull can rise rapidly if an artery leaks.

If the bleeding is from the capillaries or the veins, the blood leaks much more slowly, and the rate at which the pressure rises is slower. The slower the rise in pressure, the slower is the squeeze put on the brain, and the more slowly the symptoms and signs of the brain injury i.e., the second accident, appear.

The bleeding from blood vessels between the dura mater and the skull is most often arterial bleeding, and is called *extradural haemorrhage*, or haemorrhage on the outside of the dura mater. Because the bleeding is arterial and under pressure, the haematoma, or collection of blood, in this position can form rapidly.

The shaded section shows an extradural haematoma

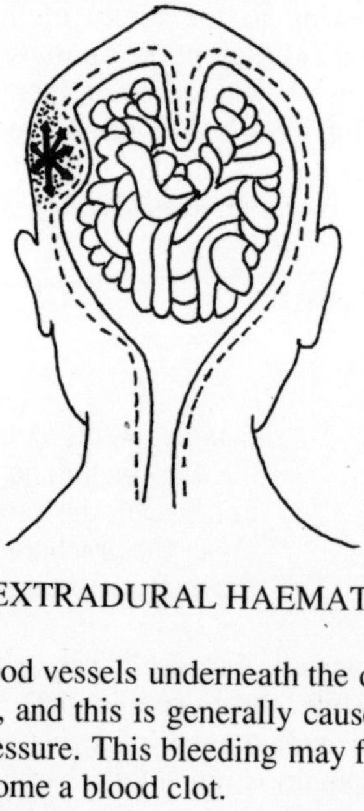

Fig. 1.5. EXTRADURAL HAEMATOMA

If the bleeding is from the blood vessels underneath the dura mater, the bleeding is called *subdural haemorrhage*, and this is generally caused by bleeding from veins or small vessels under low pressure. This bleeding may form a collection of blood, or haematoma, which can become a blood clot.

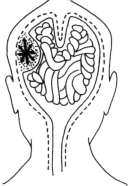

The shaded section shows
a subdural haematoma.

Fig. 1.6. SUBDURAL HAEMATOMA

If the bleeding is deeper, under the arachnoid membrane, it is called *subarachnoid*. If there is bleeding inside the brain, it is called an *intracerebral haemorrhage*, which may form an intracerebral haematoma, which may clot. *All intracerebral bleeding can produce the rise in intracranial pressure which causes the "second accident".*

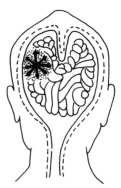

The shaded area indicates an
intracerebral haematoma.

Fig. 1.7. INTRACEREBRAL HAEMATOMA

The above information looks complicated. Draw and learn the figures. This information is worth while knowing.

33

CHAPTER 2

MEASURING THE PATIENT'S CONDITION

AND WHAT IT MEANS

The KEY WORDS in relation to measuring the patient's condition are:

COMA	unconsciousness.
GLASGOW COMA SCALE	a scale for measuring the depth of coma.
PROGNOSIS	the probable outcome of the illness.
ORIENTED	knowing where you are, who you are, who is with you, what day it is, etc.

Coma

Usually the patient with a severe brain injury is in coma. Coma means unconsciousness. Coma means that the patient does not walk, talk, or use his/her hands.

Coma may be very deep, where the patient is unrousable. In other words, nothing that you do to the patient will make him/her move, or make a noise. To find out how deeply the patient is in coma, the doctor will first of all speak to him/her to seek a response. If there is no response to voice, the doctor will squeeze hard on the finger or toenails, or will exert pressure on the neck or limbs to see if s/he will respond. Even when unconscious, s/he may still move a limb, or move the head, or make a noise in response to pain.

It is important to know if the patient is in coma, because it seems that the shorter the length of time a patient is in coma and the less deeply in coma, the better the outcome of the injury. A patient who is in coma for a long time may, however, still do well.

Glasgow Coma Scale

The standard measurement of coma is done using a scale developed by the Neurosciences Department of Glasgow University in 1974. (Graham Teasdale and Bryan Jennet, Assessment of Coma and Impaired Consciousness, A Practical Scale. *Lancet* July 13th 1974). It is now widely used, and an attempt is being made to introduce it as a universal standard for the measuring of brain injury.

On the Glasgow Coma Scale the lower the total mark is, the more severe the brain injury. The lowest total mark on the scale is 3. The highest total mark is 15. As a patient comes out of coma, the mark he gains on the scale rises. The scale is as follows:

Motor Response

obeys command	6
localizes	5
withdraws	4
abnormal flexion	3
abnormal extension	2
nil	1

Eye-opening

spontaneous	4
to voice	3
to pain	2
nil	1

Vocal Response

orientated	5
confused conversation	4
inappropriate words	3
sounds	2
nil	1

A patient with a total rating of 3, 4 or 5 is regarded as having a very severe brain injury. A person with a rating of 6, 7 or 8 has had a severe brain injury and is still in coma. A person with a rating of 9 or more may be out of coma, but still may show evidence of brain injury.

The three major factors which are measured are eye-opening, motor response and vocalization. Each of these is important, but the most important appears to be the motor response (J.Jagger, J.Jane, R.Rimel, The Glasgow Coma Scale: To Sum Or Not To Sum, *Lancet* July 9th 1983). These factors are discussed below. They are easy to understand, and you would be well advised to learn the important points of the scale.

Motor Response

The reaction of the patient to a painful stimulus may be the best indicator of the patient's condition.

Obeys = 6 points

If s/he can obey a command, when you ask him/her to do something, s/he is out of coma. You must be careful, however, that you do not "wishful think" that s/he is obeying a command. Always make sure that you have a witness for any command, so that you have someone else with whom to discuss the response.

This counts six (6) on the scale.

Also remember that sometimes these patients will obey a command when they are fresh in the morning, but they tire easily and may not obey in the afternoon. It is well to remember the fact of the approach distance also (dealt with in Chapter 6). Sometimes the patient will do nothing, if other people whom they do not know, or do not like, are in the room.

Localizes = 5 points

The term localizes means that if you cause some pain in a part of the head, limbs or body, the patient will either

1. move the hand towards that spot,
or
2. may try to push the other hand or leg towards the pain. Sometimes placing ice on the abdomen (stomach) will stimulate the patient to move a hand to push the ice away.

This counts five (5) on the scale.

Withdrawal = 4 points

The term withdrawal means that when some pain is applied to the face, or arm or leg, the patient will withdraw just that part of the body which is feeling pain away from the source of the pain.

This counts four (4) on the scale.

All of the above — obeying, localizing and withdrawing — are *local reactions*. They really indicate that the patient has a nervous system which, when stimulated, produces a local reaction and not a general reaction. To have a local reaction is much more normal than to have a general reaction to pain.

You know that if you get bitten by an ant on the foot, you may jump to start with, which is a general reaction, but then you just pull your foot away, which is a local reaction.

In other words, if your nervous system is working, it will determine the seriousness of any danger presented to it. If the danger is serious, your mind will tell your body to move totally away from the threat. If the danger is not severe, your body will conserve energy and move your limb away and not commit you to a total body movement.

Besides the local reactions discussed, there are *general reactions* or *total body reactions* which indicate a deeper or more severe degree of coma. The general reactions are two:

Abnormal flexion
Abnormal extension

Both these mean that the patient is deeply in coma.

Abnormal flexion = 3 points

With this reaction, if the stimulus of pain is applied, both arms will bend at the elbows, often the elbows will move towards each other across the body, and the wrists will bend. At the same time the legs will either straighten out or bend up.
In this reaction there is movement of all limbs. It is generalized.
This counts three (3) on the scale.

Extension = 2 points

The other generalized reaction is where the stimulus of pain is applied, the arms stretch out alongside the body, often with the palms turned away from the body and the fingers outstretched. At the same time the back of the patient may rise off the bed and the legs straighten out.
This counts two (2) on the scale.

Nil Response = 1 point

In this condition, no matter what is done to the patient, there is no response. This is the lowest point on the scale.

Eye-opening

Do not think that because the patient can open the eyes, s/he is out of coma. He may open his eyes, and still be in coma for many days or weeks.

Spontaneous = 4 points

If the patient can open the eyes spontaneously (that is, independently of a stimulus), this is good.

To voice = 3 points

If we want to wake someone who is asleep, we usually talk to them. We use a voice that is soft at first, but then we speak more loudly if we need to. Therefore, if the patient can open the eyes to someone's voice, this is a good sign, even if you have to shout.

To pain = 2 points

If a person is asleep and they do not waken when we talk to them, we usually put our hands on the person and shake them gently. If they do not waken, we often shake more roughly and might even squeeze their arm, etc. It is the same with the comatose patient. If they do not waken to voice, then the doctor will apply pain.

Nil eye-opening = 1 point

If the patient will not open the eyes to any stimulus, either to voice or pain, he receives one (1).

This inability to open the eyes may be due to:

1. Brain injury.
2. Injury to the nerves which control eye-opening.
3. Swelling around the eyes.

Pupil Size

If the pupils change their size, when a light is shone on them, and do so at a normal speed, prognosis is better than if the pupils are sluggish in movement or fixed in size and will not change when a light is shone on them.

Vocal Response

Often a patient has a tube, called an endotracheal tube in his windpipe (trachea), to help breathing, and under these conditions speech is obviously impossible.

Orientated = 5 points

If the patient knows where s/he is in regard to time and space and person, s/he is out of coma.

Confused conversation = 4 points

If the patient can say some words, even if they are incorrect, prognosis is better than if there is no speech. Confused conversation means just that. The patient can use some words, but they come out in a confused manner. It is important to realize that the words may not seem confused to the patient. S/he may know what they mean, and they will think the sentence is correct. It may be incorrect only in the way it is presented.

Inappropriate words = 3 points

If words are spoken they are not joined into sentences and are not appropriate to the circumstances.

We often find that the words that are first spoken by the patient are swear words. These often come at a moment of anger, or other intense emotion.

Sounds = 2 points

The sound may be a groan or a cry. It may be unlike any other sound that you have heard that person make. There are no formed words, but it may be an indication that an attempt is being made to communicate. Again the sounds often come when there is strong emotion emerging.

Nil vocalization = 1 point

This is the common state of the comatose patient. Most people, because of either their tracheostomy or brain injury, are unable to talk soon after the accident (except for the "Lucid Interval" which is dealt with later).

Age

In general, those who are young have a better prognosis than those who are old. The results of brain injury in people over forty are not good and those over sixty are bad. Sometimes very young children also fall into the bad-risk category.

Other important factors

If the patient's breathing, blood pressure, body temperature and body fluid control are adequate, prognosis is better than if these factors are not controlled by the body and resuscitation is required.

Coming out of coma

Some patients come out of coma quickly, within minutes of the injury, some take hours or days, and some stay in coma for weeks and months (see Fig.1.).

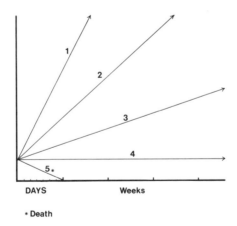

Fig. 2.1. Possible patterns of arousing from coma.

The possible patterns of patient coming out of coma are:

1. Rapid early improvement.
2. Moderate improvement.
3. Slow improvement.
4. Prolonged coma.

39

If the patient is receiving drugs, which are used to reduce the intracranial pressure, it is often impossible to judge the depth of coma accurately.

If the patient rises four levels on the Coma Scale within the first 24 hours after the injury, he has made a *rapid improvement* (see 1).

Improvement of four levels in three days would be classed as *moderate improvement* (see 2).

If the patient rises four levels on the Coma Scale in the first week after the injury, he has made a *slow improvement* (see 3).

Some patients remain on their original coma score, without change for weeks, and these are called *prolonged coma* (see 4). This is dealt with in Chapter 23.

Coma is only one sign of brain injury. It is important to understand that it is often difficult to assess the amount of brain injury that a patient has sustained until s/he has come out of coma.

Those patients who do not come out of coma, (that is are in prolonged coma) may pass into the so called "*vegetative state*"(see Chapter 23).

Mark the position of the patient as measured on the Glasgow Coma Scale on the following diagram.

DAY	1	2	3	4	5	6	7
Motor Response							
Eye Opening							
Verbal Response							
Total							

Fig. 2.2. The Patient's Glasgow Coma Scale Record.

CHAPTER 3

WHAT HAPPENS IN INTENSIVE CARE?

Usually the patient with a severe head injury is in the care of a neurosurgeon and specialists in intensive care. The neurosurgeon is a surgeon who has specialized in surgery of the brain and spinal cord.

The intensive-care specialists are often anaesthetists, or physicians, who concentrate on the care of severely injured patients. The nursing staff in this area have also had special training.

Often a patient with severe brain injury has received injury to other parts of the body. When these other injuries are serious, many doctors and nurses are involved in treatment, making sure that the patient is able to breathe properly and that the blood pressure is satisfactory, and attending to any other injuries. These matters frequently have to be dealt with before attention is given to the brain injury. Usually, the emergency treatment is carried out in the Emergency section of the hospital, and then in the Intensive Therapy Unit (I.T.U.), also known as Intensive Care Unit (I.C.U.).

No one can change the fact that some brain cells may have been killed, or severely damaged, at the time of the first accident, but everyone is very concerned that more damage may be caused by a rise in the pressure inside the skull as a result of bleeding inside the skull (intracranial haemorrhage), or swelling of the brain (cerebral oedema) i.e., the second accident. The neurosurgeon may, therefore, order special X-rays, including a C.A.T. scan.

The C.A.T. scan is a computerized X-ray of the brain, which can provide a series of pictures at different depths, and can show the brain in much greater detail than an ordinary X-ray. If there is any evidence of intracranial bleeding, or cerebral oedema, the neurosurgeon may insert through the skull, a needle attached to a tube to measure the pressure inside the skull. This instrument is called an *intracranial pressure monitor* (one type is a Richmond bolt).

If the C.A.T. scan shows that there is bleeding inside the skull, the neurosurgeon may transfer the patient to the operating theatre, to drain the blood out of the skull.

If the bleeding appears to be only a small amount, an operation may not be required, but the patient will be closely watched and may have a repeat C.A.T. scan.

If the patient has a fracture of the skull, and some of the bone has been pushed into the brain, the neurosurgeon may operate to elevate the fracture and pull the bone out of the brain. If the skull fracture is open or penetrating, the neurosurgeon may clean up the scalp and the area of injury, and remove the dead tissue and any that is severely bruised (this process is called debridement).

Sometimes, the surgeon may take a flap of bone from the skull. This may be quite large. This flap is stored under sterile conditions, and may be replaced into the skull often months later, or when the patient has recovered sufficiently.

When there is a rise in intracranial pressure (I.C.P.), owing to the swelling of the brain, surgery may not help. Control of this rise in pressure inside the skull is undertaken with the aid of drugs, and by increasing the rate of breathing of the patient (*hyperventilating*), so as to rid the blood of as much carbon dioxide as possible.

It may be that several different types of drugs need to be used in an effort to prevent or reduce a rise in the pressure inside the skull (intracranial pressure), owing to swelling of the brain (cerebral oedema).

What are all the tubes attached to the patient?

When patients are severely brain-injured, they are unable to do many of the things they would be able to do if they were conscious. Many things have to be done to keep them alive, otherwise they would die.

1. The Breathing Tube

The *endotracheal* tube, which is often as thick as a finger, goes into the mouth or nose and passes into the windpipe (trachea). This allows the patient to be attached to a machine that will breathe for him/her, called a *ventilator*. This machine can control the patient's breathing, making the breathing deeper or more shallow, or faster or slower. The machine makes sure that the patient is getting enough oxygen into his blood, while getting rid of carbon dioxide. Often, without this machine, the patient would be unable to breathe well enough and would die.

In patients who need to be ventilated for a long period, this endotracheal tube is frequently replaced by a shorter tube, which is called a *tracheostomy tube*, and which is put directly into the windpipe through the lower part of the neck. For this to be done, the patient must go to the operating theatre, to allow the surgeon to make an incision through the skin and other tissue directly into the windpipe.

2. The Feeding Tube

While food is of little importance for the few days following a severe head injury, if the patient remains in coma, or is unable to eat, a thin plastic tube, about the thickness of a pencil, is placed into the nose or mouth and inserted down into the stomach. A fluid mixture of food is fed through the tube.

3. Tubes into the Arms or Legs: The Intravenous Line

The plastic tubes going into the veins in the arms are used to provide sufficient fluid for the patient to replace fluid lost from the body through sweating, urinating and breathing. Often the brain-injured person has an imbalance occurring in the regulation of the body heat control, and becomes very hot. A lot of fluid is then lost through sweat.

These tubes are also used as an easy and painless way of giving "injections" to the patient. Through them are given such things as antibiotics to reduce infection, drugs to reduce the intracranial pressure, and drugs to relax the patient.

An intravenous line is sometimes also placed in the arm, or into the neck, which constantly monitors the pressure in the veins, thereby giving an indication of the amount of fluid in the body and how well the heart is working.

4. Tubes into the Head: The Intracranial Pressure Monitor

One tube that goes into the head passes through the scalp and the bone into cavities in the brain called the ventricles. These ventricles are full of cerebrospinal fluid, and as the pressure rises inside the skull from either a collection of blood (haematoma) or from swelling of the brain (cerebral oedema), it is transmitted to the cerebrospinal fluid. The neurosurgeon, by placing a needle through the skull into the ventricle, and therefore into the cerebrospinal fluid, can connect it to a pressure gauge (manometer), and accurately measure whether the pressure inside the brain is going up or down.

There may sometimes be other tubes in the head which are drainage tubes, draining out blood or fluid from the place where there has been damage.

5. Tube into the Bladder: The Catheter

When the patient is unconscious or very sick, s/he is unable to control the working of the bladder. A catheter, a thin tube, is inserted into the bladder to prevent it from becoming too full, and to prevent the urine leaking on to the bed. If urine does leak on to the bed, the patient is lying on a wet surface which breaks down the defences of the skin on the buttocks, and can be an important cause of infection and bedsores. It is, therefore, essential that the bladder is kept drained, so that the bed will not become wet, and the skin can remain dry. It is also important that the bladder should not be too full, because if it is constantly stretched, it will take longer to regain its ability to function. The urine output is also measured as a guide to how much fluid the patient needs.

6. Tubes in the Chest

If the patient has had a severe chest injury, thick plastic tubes may be placed through the chest wall. Air can leak through the injured site into the space between the lung and the chest wall. It may cause pressure on the lung and will make breathing difficult and also may affect the action of the heart. It therefore needs to be removed if the collection of air is too big. This removal is usually by tubes placed high in the front of the chest. If the problem is due to blood or other fluid building up inside the chest, the tubes may be placed low down in the back or side. Often a suction pump is also attached to these tubes.

Drugs

Many different drugs are used in the treatment of the patient with a severe head injury.

Some common ones are:

Antibiotics	Penicillin, ampicillin, etc., to help overcome infection.
Cortisones	Dexamethasone (Decadron), Methylprednisolone (Solumedrol), etc., to help reduce the swelling of the brain.
Relaxants	Curare, Scoline, to relax the body muscles, so that the breathing machine can work properly.
Diuretics	Lasix, Mannitol, are substances which help to remove fluid from the body and reduce the swelling in the brain.
Anticonvulsants	Dilantin, Phenobarb, Valium, are drugs that help to prevent epileptic fits.

These drugs are often given through the intravenous tube by a small attachment to that tube.

CHAPTER 4

THE THINGS THAT CAN'T BE CHANGED AND THE THINGS THAT CAN BE CHANGED

It is important for you to understand what can and can't be done in respect of your patient. It is easier to work out these things if you think of the major factors which affect the outcome of brain injury.

Some of these factors are fixed, and no one can change them in any way. Others are not fixed, and are capable of being modified; we call them non-fixed factors. You, and everyone else, can work only on the non-fixed factors.

Fixed Factors

There are two prime fixed factors. They are:

1. The severity of the primary brain injury.
2. The age of the patient.

The Severity of the Primary Brain Injury

The primary brain injury is the damage done to the brain at the time of the accident. It is the amount of brain tissue killed, or damaged, at the time of impact. Obviously if there are too many brain cells killed, or injured, the patient cannot live.

No one can be sure of the extent of the brain injury, because methods of measuring the brain are not accurate enough even to tell us the number of brain cells in a normal brain. One estimate is that there are one hundred billion brain cells in a normal brain.

It is generally accepted that once a brain cell is dead, there is no evidence that it will be replaced. It is generally thought that we have our total number of brain cells provided early in life, and that each year we lose a considerable number of them through natural wastage or injury, and that there is no reproduction or replacement of cells.

Once they are gone, they are gone and no one can change that. This concept is currently being explored and tested. If it is found that brain cells can be replaced, it will be of major significance to medicine and to people in general.

Brain injury is a fixed factor. It is also *the* most important factor. Outcome is directly related to the extent of the primary brain injury. In a severe brain injury the outcome is likely to be worse than in a milder type of brain injury.

45

It may be that much of the coma is due to injury to the part of the brain called the brainstem (see Chapter 1), some of which is reversible. The brainstem has in it the "awakening" area of the brain, and normally sends off signals to the rest of the brain to wake up. In a way, it is a bit like a car battery, which is responsible for the spark to get the motor going. Until you get the spark, the motor won't go.

It is thought that, sometimes this brainstem area is damaged and knocked out of action: really in a state of "shock". It can take time to start again, and get the rest of the brain sparking. This is what may happen to the patients who are deeply unconscious, and then apparently wake up and seem to be back to their normal self very quickly.

Unfortunately, most people think that this is what is going to happen to the person they love. This is how it is presented in the movies and on T.V. The newspapers are full of stories like the child in coma who awakens when Santa Claus enters the ward to the tune of jingle bells.

I would like to see this happen to a patient, but so far I have not been able to do so. Anyway, the main thing for you to understand is that, once a brain cell is dead, there is no evidence that it can be replaced.

The Age of the Patient

This is obviously fixed. No one can change the age of the patient and age is a significant factor in the outcome of brain injury. In general, except for babies, the younger a patient, the better the outcome.

It is certainly true that, given the same type of injury, a 20-year-old patient will do better than a 50-year-old patient, who in general will do better than a 70-year-old patient. Of course, a lot depends upon the general health of the person. A 70-year-old patient in good health may do better than a 50-year-old person who has not taken care of his/her health.

It is true, however, that a 20-year-old who has been in good health has a better chance of having a good recovery than a 50-year-old person in good health, given the same injury.

Children are different. Some of the worst head injuries occur in children, and it is difficult to predict the outcome.

Most deaths occur in the first 48 hours, and these are usually due to the enormity of the brain injury. If the person survives the first 48 hours, the next danger period appears to be at the end of the first week after the accident. Problems occur usually in the more elderly, whose heart and lungs or kidneys have difficulty coping.

The non-fixed factors

The non-fixed factors can also be split into two. It is difficult to give them a name, but I will classify them into factors relating to the

MICRO ENVIRONMENT   The Internal Affairs Department of the person.

and factors relating to the

MACRO ENVIRONMENT   The External Affairs Department of the person.

Every *country* has an External Affairs Department and an Internal Affairs Department. The External Affairs Department looks after the relationship of the country with the other countries in the world. The Internal Affairs Department looks after all the matters that relate to the running of the domestic affairs of the country.

Every *family* has an External Affairs Department, which deals with finance, banking, government matters, etc., and an Internal Affairs Department, which deals with the kitchen and the washing and the bedmaking, etc.

Every *person* has an External Affairs Department, which deals with other people and objects, etc., and an Internal Affairs Department, which keeps the body functioning. Like male and female, both departments are of equal importance.

In all the examples cited, it is important for the External Affairs and the Internal Affairs Departments to work in harmony. If only one is working properly, the other will soon deteriorate, and the country or family or person will become weak and threatened. Let us now look at these departments in the patient.

The Micro Environment: The Internal Affairs Department

All those things related to the brain function controlling the internal workings of the body we will call the Micro Environment or the Internal Affairs Department.

The brain normally keeps the body going by using its Internal Affairs Department, maintaining all normal body functions of blood pressure, breathing, eating, excretion, etc., through its nerve and hormone and muscle mechanisms.

It is very much like the work that a housewife or house husband does. Without a housewife or house husband, the home soon gets into a mess. Anyway, the plain fact is that YOU cannot be of any assistance in this housewifely duty in the brain injured.

You can't do anything about the micro environment. This is the responsibility of the medical and nursing staff in the operating theatre and in Intensive Care. They attend to all the problems involved in keeping the patient alive, stopping the bleeding in the brain, stopping the swelling of brain tissue, maintaining blood pressure and kidney function, etc.

I repeat that this is highly specialized and demanding work, which is only done by properly trained people. Obviously, this is of very high quality in any hospital that has a neurosurgery unit and an intensive care unit. You may be sure that the patient is getting the very best of care on a 24-hour basis. Without this care s/he would not survive.

The Macro Environment: The External Affairs Department

This is where you come in. Not straight away, but usually within the first ten days and with the agreement of the neurosurgeon or the director of Intensive Care. Usually by ten days, or soon after, the patient has stabilized in their Internal Affairs Department. That is most important. At this time breathing and blood-pressure controls are working, and the patient is out of the life-threatened state.

The changing problem

Now the problem changes. Unfortunately, medicine has not yet become aware of this change in the problem and tends to think that all the matters have been dealt with when the patient has a stable Internal Affairs Department.

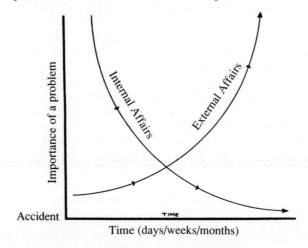

Fig. 4.1. The Changing Problem

The problem with the External Affairs Department is, however, equally important. In a way, you could say that the patient in coma has a state of *acute brain failure*. Everyone knows of acute heart failure, or acute kidney failure, or acute lung failure, but no one really thinks of acute brain failure.

Acute brain failure means that the brain cannot maintain *all* its function adequately. It may be able to look after the Internal Affairs Department, but without External Affairs the patient is in grave danger: not immediately, but in the near and the long-term future.

You can't run a house without having contact with the outside world. Every country, house or person has an External Affairs Department that must work properly.

How our brain works

What happens in the outside world has a tremendous bearing on the running of the country or house or person. Our link, as a person, into the outside world is in two ways.

We take information in and we give it out.

We take information in by our sight, hearing, touch, taste and smell. We give information out by our talking, walking and by the use of our hands. We take information in from the environment and we give it out to the environment. This is best seen as a loop:

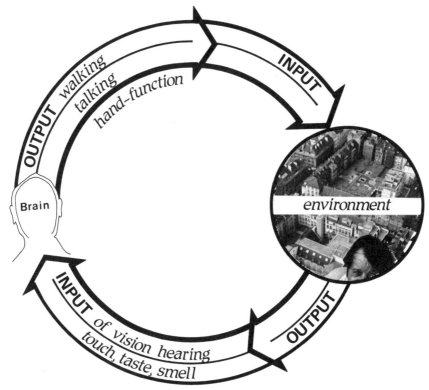

Fig. 4.2. The Cybernetic Loop

Now to take information in properly, you have to be awake. To give information out properly, you must be awake. It is the same for the patient.

THE FIRST THING WHICH MUST BE DONE FOR THE PATIENT IS TO GET HIM OR HER AWAKE.

With the patient in coma you have two choices — either:

You can wait for the patient to wake up,

or

you can see about helping him or her to wake up.

The old-fashioned idea was that coma was like being asleep, and that during the time of coma the brain was slowly healing. Some people still think this way, but they are becoming fewer. This is because it seems to be that the longer a person is in coma, the worse the outcome. In other words, people who are in coma for long periods appear to be worse off.

49

Sensory Deprivation

It may be that coma is damaging to the brain. No one has proved it, but we do know that all body tissues, no matter what, need to keep working; otherwise they slowly become weaker (atrophy).

One familiar way of looking at it is to see what happens to a person's muscles if they do not exercise them. The muscles get thinner and weaker. The same thing appears to happen to all tissue that is left without work.

You know that your brain constantly seeks and drives you to do things, whether it is going to the football or the opera, or turning on T.V. or radio, or sitting in the sun. You are all the time seeking variety, and if you don't get it, you become bored.

It has been said that "variety is not the spice of life, it is the bread of life". This could be very true. If you keep getting bored, you slowly close down and become boring. If you keep on like that, you keep decreasing your External Affairs Department and you become a hermit.

Our brains need to function by grappling with the problems of the outside world. They need information, and they get this information by the use of sight, sound, touch, taste and smell.

You also know that, if you want to become good at doing anything, you must practise it. No tennis star is at the top, unless he or she practises for many hours per day. It is the same whether you play the piano, or do any other sort of work: without constant application you will never succeed.

If you put a person in a dark hole and do not allow them to see, hear or touch anything, they are in a state called sensory deprivation. You can imagine yourself in that position. Few of us could tolerate sensory deprivation for hours, and many tests have been carried out that confirm this.

What I am suggesting is that the patient in coma is unable to pick up information from the outside world properly, because of brain injury, and is in a state of sensory deprivation. This idea is based on the work of Dr Edward Le Winn, B.S., M.D., F.A.C.P., (Director, Institute for Clinical Investigation of The Institutes for the Achievement of Human Potential, The Senior Attending Physician (Chief), Emeritus, Division of Medicine, Albert Einstein Medical Center, Philadelphia, Pennsylvania), who was a pioneer in this approach to coma.

Le Winn suggested that the place where the patient in coma is nursed can be very dangerous to him/her. It could be said that the typical ward has very little ability to give information to the patient. The patient tends to be left to wake up, with very little effort expended to make their External Affairs Department work. Le Winn suggested, therefore, that the patient was being placed in an area (the ward) which caused sensory deprivation.

You can ask yourself, "If I were placed, even fully awake, in the area where the patient is being nursed, and given the same level of input, how much would I know, or be able to do at the end of three months?" I'll bet the answer is "Not much."

Le Winn suggested that the brain-injured are deprived of normal sensory input, firstly, because they are brain-injured and, secondly, because of the environment in which they are usually placed.

You should be aware of the problem of great neglect in caring for the External Affairs Department of the patient. This area of care is not seen as true medicine by the profession and is downgraded.

This problem of neglect of the External Affairs Department of the patient is one which you can help solve. Look for it, when the patient is out of immediate danger of dying, and is being transferred from Intensive Care to the general ward, or the so-called High-Dependency ward. At this stage the neurosurgeon and the specialists in Intensive Care have done their job.

You will recognise the change very rapidly. There will not be so many nurses around as in Intensive Care, and the patient will be left much more without observation. Do not be alarmed at this. It is a good sign that the patient is out of the life-threatened state, but in a way, it is also saying that there may not be very much more offered to the patient as treatment. If you charted out how much work is being done with the patient against time, it would look like this.

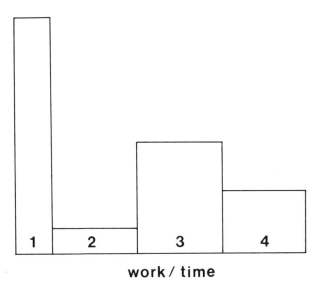

work / time

Fig. 4.3. The Amount of Work being given to the Patient
at Different Stages of Treatment.

Stage 1 shows the amount of work being done in the Accident/ Emergency wards, Operating Theatre and Intensive Care.

The drop in work input is seen in the switch to Stage 2, which is the High-Dependency ward.

Stage 3 is the change to the Rehabilitation section of the hospital, with a work increase there.

Stage 4 represents what happens when the patient is transferred home for domiciliary care.

The enormous difference in work input between Stages 1 and 2 is due to the failure of the caring professions to see the need for the External Affairs to be looked after properly.

THIS GAP IN TREATMENT CAN BE FILLED BY YOU.

Now is the time to really start waking the patient up. No one else is going to do it.

However, do not forget that when the patient does come out of coma, s/he will only then show evidence of the extent of his or her brain injury.

SECTION B

COLD BRAIN — HOT BRAIN

AND

THE APPROACH DISTANCES

The more our lives become

surrounded by the

unfamiliar and uncaring,

the more we need authentic

communication

with a few people

significant to us.

Nancy and Ernest Bormann

CHAPTER 5

THE TWO BRAINS

I remember

when my body knew

when it was time

to cry

and it was all

right then.

Bernard Gunther

We all have what amounts to two brains, in terms of human function. How they each work is of great importance to the way in which you will deal with the problem confronting you. I am not talking about the different roles of the right and left sides of the brain, although these are very important.

You have what we can call a *hot* brain and a *cold* brain. While they often work together, one is frequently dominant over the other. Both are essential to human life and activity.

You must understand that all information going into the brain has twin inputs. These twin inputs are:

1. An *objective* input. This really asks the question

"What is it?"

2. A *subjective* input. This really asks the question,

"What does this mean to me?"

How you react at any stage, in any circumstances, depends upon which of the the brains is called into use or "hooked" at that point.

Your cold brain asks the first question. Your hot brain asks the second.

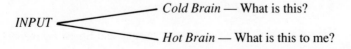

Fig. 5.1. Inputs to the brain

Just as the brain has twin inputs, one to the cold brain and one to the hot brain, it also has twin outputs. The output from the cold brain is voluntary and controls movement of the head, arms, legs, body, etc.: that is, motor action.

The output from the hot brain affects the pupils, the salivary and sweat glands, the heart and circulation, breathing, muscle tension, bowel and bladder action, etc., and is largely involuntary or automatic.

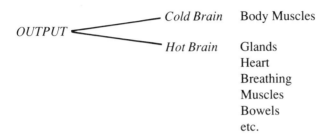

Fig. 5.2. The Cold and Hot Brain Outputs

Your hot brain, at all times, has the capacity to dominate your cold brain, unless you can control it. You have seen people whose hot brain is in action. You have felt what it is like yourself.

The hot brain is thus our emotional brain. It is much more spontaneous and primitive than our cold brain, and it can dominate the cold brain very effectively. It can literally swamp our cold brain. That is why we talk about a person who loses their temper as having "lost their cool", or we say to them "Don't get all hot and bothered about it."

We have all felt our hot brain in action when we are suddenly put in a difficult position. We feel our heart thumping in our chest, our mouth goes dry, we start to breathe more rapidly, our muscles feel tighter and we feel uneasy in the abdomen. These feelings are normal if we strike trouble, and they move us to get into action, deciding either to go away from the problem, or fight it, or try to delay what is occurring i.e, the "fight or flight" reaction.

You have all felt your hot brain in action at some time. No doubt you felt all these hot-brain things when you first received the message that an accident had happened to a member of your family. A common feeling is that "my legs turned to jelly", or "I was a quivering mass." This is your hot brain dominating your reactions. It is a normal feeling, when we are overwhelmed by something that appears to be outside our ability to control.

Your cold brain would then assert itself, and you would begin to ask questions about the accident. Once you found that your son or daughter was still alive, you would feel some relief, and your next question would be directed to finding out how severe was the damage, and where the patient was.

All this information goes into your cold brain. If you are overwhelmed again by the gravity of the situation, your hot brain will once more come into action, and you may start to cry.

If you can't get satisfactory answers, and your hot brain continues to dominate, you will become tense, your heart will throb again, and all the symptoms of hot brain activity will recommence. This move into the hot brain occurs normally and can go on for days. You need to cry, whether you are a "macho" man or a "liberated" woman. It is part of your natural method of coping with stress.

But after hours or days, depending on your personality, the cold brain needs to take over. If you remain dominated by your hot brain, you will be ineffective just when you need to function effectively. If your hot brain stays in control, you will go round in circles mulling over what has occurred, without moving forward to deal with the problem. It is very much like a motor car with its engine running, being "revved up" in neutral. It makes a loud noise and uses a lot of energy, but it is unproductive. It does not move forward.

Your cold brain is needed to deal with the reality of the problem, to put your whole brain into gear and to move forward. The problem now is "to where" and "how"?

Your cold brain needs facts, accurate information, so that it can make judgments and plan effective action. It needs you to know where you are going. You still feel that you are "lost", and no one can feel that way without their hot brain reacting.

The only way to move from hot brain to cold brain is to get the facts, and consider what you should do with them. So let's start off with what these facts are likely to be. There is only one answer. They will be bad. This is a catastrophe. Any severe brain injury is a catastrophic event.

Within the first few days death is always a strong possibility, but as the days go by it becomes less likely. Most deaths occur within the first 48 hours, and then there is a rapid decrease in the numbers who die after that time. This applies particularly with young adult patients, who have enormous powers of survival. Certainly, by the end of the first week most of those patients who are going to die will have done so.

> No one can tell you how long a severely brain-injured person will stay in coma. If the patient comes out of coma rapidly, the possibility of recovery is greater than when the patient stays in coma for a long time.

"The only question I want to ask, you can't answer. No one can." This was the way one mother answered me when I spoke to her about her brain-injured son in coma. I had asked her if she had any questions, and that was her reply. She was right. She wanted to know how long it would be before her son would come out of coma. No one could tell her.

That kind of non-information is no good for your cold brain. It is even worse for your hot brain. We all see coming out of coma as a bench-mark. It is the first thing that needs to happen, if a patient is to recover. Everyone is afraid that the person whom they love will remain in prolonged coma. We have all read about such cases in the newspapers, and the thought fills us with horror.

It is worth remembering that most patients do indeed come out of coma, and that only a small percentage go into prolonged coma: that is, for a period of weeks or months. It is also important to realize that when the patient does come out of coma, there may be evidence of severe brain injury that is sufficient to prevent normal functioning in almost any manner, and which may even lead to total dependence on care for a lifetime.

What you have to do is obtain as much information as possible about what should be done, so that you can get your cold brain working and limit the amount of hot-brain input, to see what you can do for the patient.

The way you feel can be diagrammed like this.

PROBLEM

If you go down the Hot Brain track you will notice;

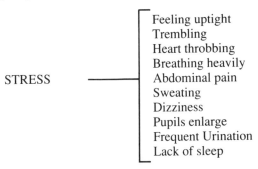

All these symptoms will make you feel worse, and more worried and increase the amount of stress. You will then feel uptight again, and the whole process will turn into a vicious cycle. If you continue on this track, you will begin to have symptoms of extreme stress. You can't help going down this track for a while. No one is totally cold brain, and if disaster has struck you, you will react with your hot brain.

If the hot brain continues in control, that is where the danger lies. It would be wise for you to go to someone for advice on how to deal with this stress. There are also books easily available that could be helpful.

If you go down the Cold Brain track, you will:

1. Seek accurate information.
2. Confirm its accuracy and its relevance to your problem.
3. Assess what action should be taken.
4. Work out how to take the correct action.
5. Constantly monitor the effect of the action.
6. Change the action, if it becomes inappropriate.
7. Monitor the change.

You will need your diary to help you do all of this. You will also require constant information from those who are looking after the patient.

So you must go on to the cold brain track. Your cold brain is your logical brain. Being logical, it must search for answers. To get answers, it must have *information*.

Without information, you cannot plan your actions, and if you cannot plan your actions in this disaster, it becomes more difficult to find your way through the system.

Barbara Brown in *Super Mind* (Harper Row, Bantam Books, New York 1980) writes: "The role of information for the person under stress is paramount for his relief . . . The only reason for unproductive problem-solving and stress is lack of information."

The primary place to get your information is from those who are looking after the patient: the doctors and nurses. As I said before, expect them to tell you the truth. If they do not know what the likely outcome is, that is what they will say. If you have any doubts about what is being said, then you must ask them to explain more carefully. You will find this book a useful guide in your approach to them.

CHAPTER 6

THE APPROACH DISTANCE

You do not transgress

over this line

with impunity.

Introduction

Your first impression may be that this is not a very important chapter. You would be wrong. It is one of the most important chapters in the book, and you will need to understand it well if you are to attempt to protect the patient you love from the hurts of the world.

We are all territorial animals, and we guard our territory very closely. All countries have territorial limits, which they do not like violated. The country controls not only its land mass, but also its air space and its coastal borders, even miles out to sea. Any intruder needs to be identified as friend or enemy, and dealt with accordingly.

In our own countries, if we hear that there is repeated violent crime in another city, we may think how unfortunate that is. If the repeated violence is in our own city, we are more concerned. If we hear that the violence is in our own suburb, then the worry becomes greater. If it is in our street, it becomes more worrying for us. If it is in our own house, then it is a major concern.

We are all territorial animals. Just as a dog guards his territory, we guard ours. We all have an approach distance for everything, which we develop from childhood and even from infancy.

The Approach Distances

There are actually two different approach distances, but we work them as one. These approach distances are;

1. How close do we approach other people, or animals or objects.
2. How close do we allow other people, or animals or objects, to approach us.

The First Approach Distance

Let me take the matter of us approaching other people. You probably know people whom you do not like terribly much, and whom you avoid as much as possible. If you see them coming towards you in the street, you may make an attempt to move out of their path, or even hide in a shop doorway. You are setting your approach distance to them.

It is the same when you are with animals. Some people are frightened of dogs, and will not go near them. You may not be frightened of dogs, but you are probably more confident about approaching a small dog such as a Dachshund rather than a big dog such as an Alsatian. If the dog has a reputation for being savage, such as some Alsatians or Dobermans, you will be even more careful about how closely you move towards them.

Your approach distance will be greater if, for instance, the dog is a Doberman showing its teeth, growling and straining on a leash. You will stay clear, unless you know the dog. If there is a strong mesh fence between you and the animal, your approach distance will become shorter, and you may walk up to within centimetres of it, even if it is growling and displaying its teeth. You change your approach distance instinctively, depending upon the threat or possible threat to you.

The same reaction occurs with objects. If you like rock-climbing, you may approach the edge of a cliff without any worries, and your approach distance becomes so short that you may climb down it and enjoy doing it. Someone who dislikes cliffs, however, will stay away from the edge for fear of falling.

The blind person uses a white stick, not only to signify that he is blind, but taps along the street detecting the pavement and obstacles, to measure the approach distance of both objects and people to himself.

The mother who tells her son to move away from the fire, or to look both ways at the kerbside, is teaching him approach distances.

We are all the same. We constantly guard our approach distance from people, animals and objects.

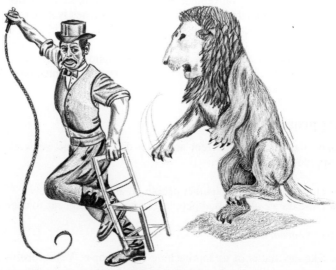

Fig. 6.1. Maintaining the Approach Distance

60

The Second Approach Distance

We constantly guard how close we let people, animals or objects come to us.

As I said, we stay away from people whom we do not like. In general, the only people we will allow to touch us in any way are those close to us, with whom we are on very friendly terms i.e, a friend or relative. In general, we will not let others touch us, and will withdraw from them if they attempt to do so.

The same thing applies with animals. If we feel threatened by an animal, if a dog or a horse rushes towards us, we will attempt to move out of its way. We will withdraw and maintain our approach distance.

It also applies with objects. When driving along a highway, if a large vehicle comes into the space behind you, you will note it very quickly because of its size. If the driver moves close to you, you may become uncomfortable, and if s/he "rides on your back bumper-bar", the closeness may become unbearable for you, and you may decide to pull off the road and let him/her pass.

Personal Space

We all have this approach distance for all things. It has been called "personal space" and likened to a "space bubble" which we all have around us. Allan Pease (*Body Language, signals; How to Use Body Language for Power, Success and Love*, Camel Publishing Company, 1981) has set out some common approach distances for middle-class people living in developed countries. He sets four zones, moving from the body outwards.

1. *The Intimate Zone*: the bubble which surrounds us to a distance of 45 cm. (18 in.). Even in this zone there are subzones, depending upon the part of the body concerned.

Desmond Morris in *Manwatching* (Jonathan Cape, Great Britain, 1977) refers to them as taboo zones. He says, "In general, as might be expected, the body zones nearest to sexual features showed the strongest taboos and those furthest away showed the weakest."

2. *The Personal Zone*: the bubble which is around us at a distance of between 46 cm. and 1.22 m. (18 to 48 in.). This is the general range into which we allow friends.

3. *The Social Zone*: the bubble which is around us at a distance of between 1.22 m and 3.6 m (4 to 12 feet). This is the distance at which we negotiate with people.

4. *The Public Zone*: the area outside our social zone (over 3.6 m (12 feet), which is the distance at which we stand when addressing a group of people.

Many people would now say that we also have another distance, our *inner space*, which is totally under our control and into which no person can venture without our express permission. In my experience there are times when I assume that the so-called vegetative patient retreats into her/his inner space, to allow survival amidst the onslaughts of the hostile environment into which s/he is so often deposited.

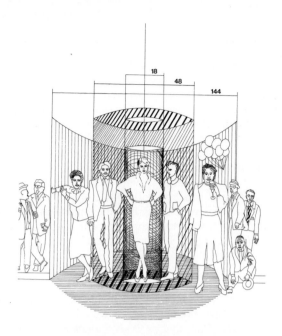

Fig. 6.2. Diagram of Personal Spaces

Threats to Personal Space

What Happens When our Personal Space is Threatened

The closer we come to being threatened by people, or things, or objects, the more our own "personal space" is likely to be violated (the same as a country's air or land or sea space is by an intruder), and we need to take action.

The action we take can be one of four different manoeuvres, or a combination of them. We can:

1. Use a facial expression.

or

2. Use our voice, either to tell the threatening object to go away, to leave us alone, or call for help.

or

3. Use our hands and arms to defend ourselves, either by punching or by using a weapon, such as a club, spear, gun, etc.

or

4. We can use our legs to move us away from the violating object or person (that is, we can "clear out").

In other words, we go through our primitive "fight or flight" routine. It should be once again stated that not only does the "fight or flight" get our cold brain working to deal with the problem, it also gets our hot brain working with all the effects on:

our skin,	with sweating and shivering;
on our muscles,	which tighten up;
on our pupils,	which get bigger;
on our throat,	which becomes dry;
on our breathing,	which become more rapid;
on our heart,	which starts to thump and beat faster;
on our bowels,	which want to move;
on our bladder,	which wants to empty.

These are indications that we are aroused and ready to fight or flee.

Suppose we cannot fight or flee, that we are unable to use our voice or our hands or our feet. Suppose that we are bound and gagged. We are at the mercy of some threat and the situation becomes intolerable for us. If we cannot get help, the only way out for us is to withdraw mentally into our inner space, from the reality of what is happening, and sink into a state of apathy (in other words "give up"), or else we can become mentally unbalanced.

How the Brain-injured's Personal Space is Threatened

Now let us consider the person who is brain-injured, lying in a hospital bed. We see him/her with intimate space violated, the personal bubble broken into by a tracheotomy tube intruding into the throat, a nasogastric tube intruding into the nose, a catheter intruding into the bladder, and often an intravenous drip intruding into the veins of the arm. S/He often has monitor leads from an electrocardiograph attached to the chest, and s/he is hooked up to a selection of machines. S/He often has a plaster cast on one or more limbs, s/he is unable to talk and often unable to move his or her head, shoulders, arms, trunk and legs.

When the person is deeply in coma, we can assume that s/he has no concept of body space, or that his/her personal space is being violated. As consciousness returns, as s/he comes out of the coma, and awareness is increasing, his or her body image may be being restored, and so is the desire to protect and safeguard his/her body space. S/He most certainly will have no recall about how he came to be in this frightening position, but in a blurred way s/he may know that the people who performed all these terrible intrusions into the body space are the ones who surround him or her most of the time.

Why the Brain-injured's Personal Space Is Threatened

1. All the tubes, leads, drips that are inserted into, or attached to, the patient are there for a purpose. They are all part of the measures which medicine uses to help to keep the patient alive, and to get them through the acute stage of the injury.

Without these aids, and the knowledge which goes with them, the chances of survival of the patient would be very small, if not impossible. They are a necessary intrusion into the intimate space.

2. While to you there is only one person in the hospital who matters, the medical and nursing staff and the paramedical staff have many other patients to whom they must attend. Your thoughts and eyes are focused on one person. They must deal with, and treat, many.

You will have already noticed the intense care which is given to the patient in the Intensive Therapy Unit. If s/he has been moved from the unit to another ward, you will have noticed that there is a great reduction in the number of staff available.

It is a fact of hospital life that Intensive Therapy Units are very well staffed, but as a patient is moved from there along the hospital chain towards discharge or transfer, the number of staff becomes less per patient.

The hospital and the State cannot afford to provide staff for all parts of the hospital in the same numbers as in the Intensive Therapy Unit. Nor is this necessary. It would, in most cases, be a great waste of human resources.

This fact is no help to you, or the patient, if s/he needs more than the hospital can provide. If the hospital cannot provide the staff you need, then it must come from another source (that is, you, your family and friends).

3. Teaching hospitals are acute hospitals. This means that they like to deal with the patient who has a sudden illness or accident. They have to try to keep their beds available for patients who suffer sudden illness or accident. If they let the beds of the hospital become full of long-term patients, there is no room for the acutely ill.

In general, the staff are accustomed, therefore, to caring for patients who come in for a short period of time, who get treated, and who get better. Like all people, the caring professions like to see the results of their work in as short a time as possible. While most patients who are acutely ill get better fairly quickly and are therefore seen as a "win", the patients with severe brain injury take a long time and are often seen as "no win". They are not as welcome as other patients from a psychological point of view.

4. Often the caring professions see the patient who is severely brain-injured as a non person. They are involved with communication with the patient, used to asking the question, "How are you feeling today?" and obtaining a reply. If no reply comes, the inference is that the person is deaf, or does not understand the question and is therefore mentally abnormal, in which case s/he is incapable of correct thought.

Conclusion

So much of our civilisation depends upon speech. It is often through speech that a judgment is made on the "intelligence" of a person. When the patient still has a tracheotomy tube in place; s/he is unable to talk, or to make any sound, and so in the frame of thinking which the caring professions have been taught, the patient is seen as incapable of thought. This impression is confirmed when it is seen that the patient also has a nasogastric tube intruding into the nose and a catheter intruding into the bladder, for no normal-intelligence person would put up with such a state.

The whole message being sent to the doctor or nurse or physiotherapist or occupational therapist is that the patient is a non-person. That is how the patient is often treated. (This statement is a generalisation. Many members of the caring professions identify that the patient is a person even in these circumstances.)

The tragedy is that this "non-person" attitude with its consequent actions, besides being unnecessary, is not a deliberate attempt on the part of the caring professions to treat the patient as a non-person. It is produced by thoughtlessness or rather non-thinking, by ignorance.

I recall seeing a patient who, for 11 months, had had a tracheotomy tube in place, was being fed through a nasogastric tube, had her right hand tied to the bed to stop her pulling out the tubes, and was regarded as being still in coma. After I had spoken to the relatives and nursing staff and filled in the questionnaire, it became obvious to me that she was out of coma.

I sent her husband into the room to tell her that I was coming to see her, and when I walked in, she had an adoring look on her face as her husband spoke to her. I introduced myself and told her that I would not hurt her, and that I would tell her every time I was going to touch her (that is, every time I was going to intrude into her intimate space), and when I requested her to move her right toes, she did so. When I requested her to move her left toes, she did so. I questioned how could she be in coma, when she could obey a command.

I asked them to get her out of bed, sit her up, start to put something she liked on to her tongue to give her the taste of food, see about getting her tracheotomy out, and giving her a proper bath. I then laid out a correct programme for her. For almost a year she had been surrounded by loving, caring people, but they did not know what to do. In this case it was not their attitude which was faulty, but their knowledge.

The people who see the patient most as a person are the relatives and friends. They have no doubt that the patient remains the centre of their love and affection, even with all the tubes intruding and in such a threatening environment. So the patient is dependent upon those who love him/her to safeguard his/her approach distance. If they do not, it is unlikely that anyone else has either the time or the attitude to do so.

CHAPTER 7

SAFEGUARDING THE APPROACH DISTANCE

FOR THE PATIENT

"What is believed to be essential for mental health is that the infant and young child should experience a warm, intimate and continuous relationship with his mother (or permanent mother substitute) in which both find satisfaction and enjoyment."

John Bowlby, *Attachment*
(Pelican Books 1972)

Within each of us is the child. Within each of us is the child who needs security and comfort. Within the person who is brain injured, this need may become of paramount importance.

In the Introduction I wrote how it feels to be lost; lost in a system which you can't control. The patient is in the same position: in a lost situation and desperately seeking to find a way back to normality. It has been said, "It is very much like being at the bottom of a swimming-pool, and looking up towards the surface through the water. Everything is vague and obscured and unreal."

What the patient needs most is YOU: your involvement and time. The presence of someone they love and is familiar to them. They need their guide with the map to bring them from their lost state back on the road to normality. They need you to treat them as a person, to protect them from the indignities they suffer as a patient, to spend time with them and to fill them with your love.

If you look at the fact that the patient is in the hospital for 24 hours every day, surrounded by busy, transient nursing and medical staff, it will be obvious that he or she has no one to link on to: to give security while they are separated from family and friends.

Someone will have to spend 8-10 hours each day with the patient to provide the security they need. The comfort of a friendly presence is especially important in the early stages, until the patient comes out of coma. This is essential. Your presence will be needed for a long period of time, for s/he is in a heavily threatening environment.

You also need to establish protection and safeguards while you are not present. You must make up a NOTICE with big printed letters at least 5 cm high. Make it in red on a yellow piece of cardboard and place it above the bed.

On it you will put:

Name . . . . is severely brain-injured.

He (She) is in coma. However, he (she) may be able to see or hear or feel you.
Would you please identify yourself to him (her).
Would you please

1. Not say anything which is negative in his (her) presence.
2. Not laugh at anything he (she) does.
3. Tell him (her) if you are going to touch him (her).
4. Tell him (her) where you are going to touch him (her).
5. Tell him (her) what you are going to do.
6. Talk to him (her) as a person.
7. Talk to him (her) slowly, in a loud, clear voice.
8. If there are more than one of you, do not all talk together.
9. Praise him (her), if you think there has been a response to you.
10. Say that he (she) is going to get better, and that you are going to help him (her).

Every day when you are there, you should feed positives into the patient. Tell them that they are going to get better, even if you are not sure that they can hear you.

Stroke them with your hands when they are unsettled and agitated, and talk to them at the same time.

The majority of patients I have seen in coma will respond when a close member of the family, or a friend, talks to them and strokes them when they are upset.

This was demonstrated very vividly with one patient called Paul. His hot brain was so active when he was moved out of intensive care that he was sweating profusely, trembling with his arms outstretched, wide-eyed and staring with his hair almost standing up. It was extremely worrying to see him so, and there were indications that he would need to be sedated with a lot of drugs.

His mother went in and spoke to him and stroked him and told him that he would be all right, and within minutes he settled down. This same scene occurred frequently over a period of weeks. Each time his mother was successful in comforting and settling him down. Other people also tried, when his mother was not available, but they were not as successful.

He was an extreme case but we have seen the same results repeated with many patients at many times. It appears to be that, in some intangible way, the "vibes" that pass between people who love each other are still present, even if the patient looks to be in coma.

A similar indication of this occurred with a child in an intensive care ward. The Coma Arousal head nurse pointed this out in a major teaching hospital. She had commenced on the programme of visual and auditory stimulation with the child, a girl of 7. The child's heart rate went up to 140. When the mother of the child took over and did the same things, the child's heart rate went down to the 90s, indicating that she had settled. (This would lend itself well to a defined study).

How the patient attempts to guard approach distance

Once the patient starts to come out of the coma, and especially once movement of some part of the limbs or body returns, s/he will attempt to safeguard their own personal space or bubble. They will use the same three methods that we normally use: speech, arm movement, or leg movement. They will:

1. Make a noise to attract your attention or to complain. This is unlikely to be in words until they are a long way down the road to recovery.
2. They will move one or both arms.
3. They will move their legs.

It is most unlikely that these movements will be co-ordinated. They will appear random and repetitive and to have no purpose. They will often be accompanied by a tremor or shaking.

What The Patient May Do with Intruding Devices

With their arms they may move their hand towards the nasogastric tube in the nose, or to the tracheostomy tube in the neck, or to the catheter into the bladder. It is as if they are saying through body language, "I want these things out of my own intimate, personal space." They will often try to hook them out. Even if they cannot use their fingers to grasp, they may hook their hand around them and pull.

What the Patient May Also Do

To safeguard themselves generally, they may do the following:

1. Their facial expression may show dislike or anger.
2. If they can, they may start to groan or cry or shout in fear or anger. (One of the classic demands was from a 16-year-old girl who got her speech back early, and on surveying her left arm in plaster said, "Who will take this shitting thing off my arm!")
3. They may start to resist people doing things to them. They may push people away or try to strike them.
4. They may try to move their body out of the bed or out of the chair.

They are demonstrating through their body language that their intrinsic drive to get better is becoming stronger. They are saying that they do not like what has happened to them, or what people are doing to them. They are saying that they want "out".

Unfortunately, because patients are seen as non-persons, as a person who could not possibly have a brain working, many of these attempts to express themselves will be seen as "bad" by the caring professions. Hospitals are orderly places. The best patients are seen to be those who behave themselves, rarely ring the bell for attention, eat correctly, speak nicely to the doctor and nurses, never move without being asked, show proper respect for the system which is helping them, take their drugs without any fuss, have their bowels open every day, and go to sleep at night at the correct time.

The brain-injured patient, coming out of coma, does none of these things. They are seen as a great trouble. Not only that, they are seen as a great trouble for a long time. They are not just going to be unpleasant for a few days. They are going to be unpleasant for many months, and there is no guarantee that it will all be worth it.

The brain-injured person is an anathema to the hospital system. Therefore the things that are likely to happen will be:

1. They will be sedated. They will be given a tranquillising drug, which will have the effect of putting them back into a coma. (I have seen several patients sedated heavily back into a comatose state.)

2. They will be restrained. The arm or leg which can move will be tied to the bed or to the chair. They will be made chairfast or bedfast. If more than one limb is moving, or they are moving from a chair, they may be girdled around with one or more sheets tying them to the chair.

As has been commented in my presence, Amnesty International would be contacted if this close restraint were exercised on political prisoners.

What to do

While the patient is incapable of protecting his or her personal space, you actually have a great deal of power. You may need to pluck up your courage, and exert your authority as the next of kin and seek explanation of all that is done. You will, of course, be seen as difficult by the hospital staff, but the benefits far outweigh the potential losses.

Ask about sedation, restraint, tubes and inhibition plasters in the following manner:

1. Sedation

Recognize that sometimes patients need sedating, but this should be the minimum quantity for the shortest time. Ask:

1. What drug is being given?
2. What are the effects likely to be?
3. What are the side effects of the drug?
4. Does it interact with other drugs the patient is on ?
5. How long is it likely to be required?
6. Will the drug be monitored?
7. What will be the factors which indicate that the patient can come off the drug?
8. Who will make the decision to stop the drug?

While you must be guided by the medical staff and take their advice, it is often preferable for you to ask if you can stay with the patient and help to settle her or him down rather than that heavy sedation should be resorted to.

2. Restraint

Some patients are restrained. That means their arms or legs or body are tied to a chair or to a bed. This applies often to the patients who are most mobile, and staff are worried about their falling from the bed or from the chair. Their worry is legitimate. They are legally responsible for the care of the patient. They do not have enough staff to watch the patient constantly, and if a patient does fall out of bed, the matter is considered very seriously from a legal point of view and reported to the administration of the hospital. One way to help overcome this problem is to ask if he or she can be put on a mattress on the floor. The ward sister can usually do this on her own authority. Some will gladly agree. Others will feel that it makes the room look "messy".

One way for you to help is to volunteer your presence for the first few times, so that all have the comfort of your presence.

3. Tubes

If the patient is trying to pull out tubes, question if they still really need to be used. Ask:

1. How much longer are the tubes likely to be required?
2. What will be the factors which indicate that the patient can have the tubes out?
3. Who will make the decision to take the tubes out?
4. In regard to the nasogastric tube, ask if the patient is yet fit to start taking food orally. If so, ask if you can be shown the correct way to feed him or her. (Most mothers who have fed their babies are very adept at feeding a person coming out of coma.)

4. Inhibition Plasters

Be careful with a plaster of Paris put on the limbs. The general approach is that it is to prevent the limbs from contracting up. This may or may not be effective. Certainly it gives the caring professions the feeling that they are doing something positive, but remember that placing a limb in a plaster cast stops movement of the limb and that may be bad. Many hospitals do not use them. I believe that they make things more difficult for the patient, especially if the patient is trying to get some movement in the limb and s/he has the additional weight of the plaster to shift as well. I believe that there are times when this additional weight is sufficient to stop spontaneous movement and slow down the recovery of the patient.
Ask:

1. Why are casts being used?
2. How effective are they?

3. Is there any scientific evidence that this is so?
4. Who will decide when the cast should be removed?

All these questions can be put pleasantly to the appropriate doctors. If you feel you would have difficulty obtaining this information, then write to the doctor and ask for it. If you cannot obtain a reply, seek the help of your family doctor or the Medical Administrator in charge of the hospital. Most doctors will gladly provide the information you want, but you need to ask them.

ACTION SHEET

1. ACKNOWLEDGE THAT YOU HAVE HOT BRAIN WORKING. IF YOU CANNOT SLOW IT DOWN, SEEK SOME PROFESSIONAL HELP OR SPIRITUAL HELP FROM YOUR CLERGY, OR HELP FROM YOUR FRIENDS.

2. SEEK THE INFORMATION REFERRED TO IN SECTION A. REMEMBER YOUR COLD BRAIN NEEDS INFORMATION.

3. UNDERSTAND THE IDEA OF PERSONAL SPACE. IDENTIFY THE WAYS IN WHICH THE PERSONAL SPACE OF THE PATIENT IS VIOLATED.

4. IDENTIFY THE WAYS IN WHICH THIS INTRUSION INTO PERSONAL SPACE CAN BE REDUCED AND DISCUSS THESE WITH THE DOCTOR.

5. MAKE UP THE CHART TO GO OVER THE BED. EMPHASIZE THAT THE PATIENT IS A PERSON WHO IS VALUABLE TO YOU.

6. IF AGGRESSION OCCURS, SEEK TO HAVE IT IDENTIFIED AS A SIGNIFICANT STEP FORWARD FOR THE PATIENT. TAKE MEASURES TO REDUCE THE AGGRESSION BY YOUR PRESENCE.

7. CHECK ON DRUG THERAPY AND ASKED TO BE NOTIFIED OF ANY ADDITIONAL DRUGS GIVEN TO THE PATIENT.

8. IF RESTRAINT IS NEEDED, EITHER FOR THE SAFETY OF THE PATIENT, OR THE STAFF, SEEK WAYS TO REDUCE THE INTENSITY OR DURATION OF THE RESTRAINT.

9. WITH ALL TUBES INSERTED INTO THE PATIENT'S BODY, ACKNOWLEDGE THAT THEY ARE NECESSARY, BUT SEEK THEIR REMOVAL AT THE EARLIEST TIME.

10. IF YOU FAIL TO OBTAIN WHAT YOU WANT IN ONE WAY, DO NOT CAUSE ANTAGONISM, BUT SEEK AN ALTERNATIVE PATHWAY.

SECTION C

ASSESSING THE PATIENT

More things are missed

by not looking

than

by not knowing.

Old medical axiom.

CHAPTER 8

IS THE PATIENT STILL IN COMA?

"Just as an explorer penetrates into

new and unknown lands, one makes discoveries

in the every day life,

and the erstwhile mute surroundings

begin to speak a language which becomes

increasingly clear."

W. Kandinsky, *Point and Line to Plane*,
(Solomon Guggenheim Foundation 1947)

You will be exploring into new and unknown lands, the mute surroundings will speak and the language will become increasingly clear. While Kandinsky wrote about art, the same applies to all areas of human endeavour.

You must first find out if the patient is still in coma. In Chapter 2, you will have read about the Glasgow Coma Scale. That scale is useful for measuring the patient in coma soon after the injury, but it is not of great value when the patient is coming out, or should be coming out, of coma.

You need to know if the patient is still in coma, and if so, what type. The time to make this judgment is usually when the patient has been moved to a high dependency ward. This move really means that the hospital accepts as fact that the patient can do nothing for himself or herself, and is totally dependent on other people for care. This is where your work begins in earnest.

You already know that to leave a patient in coma might be dangerous for them. You already know that medicine does not offer very much apart from keeping the Internal Affairs Department of the patient working. You already know that the involvement of the medical profession has dropped dramatically. You already know that there is a big change in the number of nursing staff who are looking after the patient. You already know that the paramedical departments of physiotherapy and occupational therapy have little time to spend with the patient. You already know that your special person has not yet reached a level of function which would be acceptable to you, nor would it be acceptable to him or her.

Perhaps you already have been told that the outlook is very grim and that there is really no chance of doing anything further to help. You already know that the caring professions have consigned your person to the irretrievable basket or to the poor prognosis classification.

You already know that the social work department is beginning to tell you that you must start the grieving process, which will lead on to the acceptance of this disastrous state.

You know all these things. They are fed into you and your cold brain registers them. You know all these things, but you refuse to accept them. Your hot brain says "NO! NO! NO! NO!"

You will be told that this refusal to accept is part of the grieving process. You will be told that you will come to accept the reality (as seen by other people) in time, and that you should direct your energies to accept *their* imposed reality. What everyone is inferring or may be saying to you, is, "Things are looking bad. Not much can be done. We must wait and see what happens."

You are saying to yourself, "They are the experts. But I love my son, daughter, wife, husband, father or friend. How can I give up?"

Well, you must be realistic. The odds against anyone coming back to a useful productive life after severe brain injury are small in orthodox medicine.

Dr A Bricolo and his colleagues, in 1980 reported in the *Journal of Neurosurgery*,(*J. Neurosurgery*, 52: 625 -634, 1980) the outcomes for 135 patients in coma for two weeks caused by brain injury, and of those patients one year after injury: (see Chapter 24)

30% had died

40% were vegetative or severely disabled

17% had made a moderate recovery, meaning that they were independent but disabled

13% had made a good recovery, possibly implying they were capable of resuming normal life.

Dr Bricolo and his colleagues make some very interesting points about these results. He writes " . . . it makes it mandatory to continue rehabilitation relentlessly in all cases", and "What makes the final balance sheet so dismaying is . . . the high incidence of outcomes implying severe disablement and making the survivors totally dependent on others and capable of suffering and grief. We are prepared to admit that this may be due also or even prevalently to the inadequacy of rehabilitation therapy."

What to do?

You can do nothing. Freeze in fright. Let your hot brain run. Accept the inevitable.

OR

You can attempt to help the person you love back to life.

You may not succeed. It is unlikely that you will ever get them back to where they were. They will be different. So will you, of course. No one can go through this experience as a patient or as a relative, and not be different from before.

You don't know where the end point of recovery will be. You do not know how far along the path to normality you will get the patient. You may not succeed in achieving anything, or you may succeed in achieving something far beyond your wildest dreams.

It depends upon your philosophy; on how you think and feel about it all. If you are like those relatives and friends with whom we deal, you have no choice. You will go ahead.

Richard Bergland has written in *The Fabric of the Mind* (Penguin Books 1985), "As a bystander, it appears to me that the human mind, in its darkest hours, seeks the brightest guiding star. It seems to thrive on the conversion of problems to opportunities."

This is my experience also. Almost without exception, when people are given the opportunity to do something, even without any guarantee that it will work, they will grasp that opportunity.

If you are going to grapple with the problem, you have to concentrate on the areas which concern you.

I have already said that you can't do anything about the primary brain injury (the injury caused at the time of the accident) or the age of the patient, and that these factors are fixed and inflexible.

I have already said that the neurosurgeons and the Intensive Care staff are experts in keeping the body alive and attending to the Internal Affairs of the patient.

I have already said that the External Affairs Department of the person is sadly neglected by all, and that it is of great importance for all of us, to allow us, to deal with the environment.

Remember the loop mechanism again. Remember the way in which we relate to the world. Remember we need our sight, hearing, touch, taste and smell so we can take in information about the world and our immediate environment so we know "what goes on". We need our motor actions to allow us to respond to the world and give it a stimulus from us.

Your first job

Your first job is to find out the conscious state of the patient. Strange as it may seem, there is a lot of confusion as to when a patient is out of coma.

All of us know that, if we are talking to someone and they indicate that that they are aware that we are talking to them, even if they do not understand the content of the talk or what it means, then we both must be awake and aware and not in coma.

We really do depend upon the other person sending us signals through voice or action, which we can pick up and respond to. Body language through facial expression or body position can tell us so much.

The whole of our living depends upon our ability to pick up information and change our environment, or position in that environment. Once again we come back to the cybernetic loop, which is a Stimulus-Response loop.

The patient who has been brain-injured may have only one part of the loop working: that is, he may be able to receive the stimulus but not make a response.

This can be shown diagrammatically:

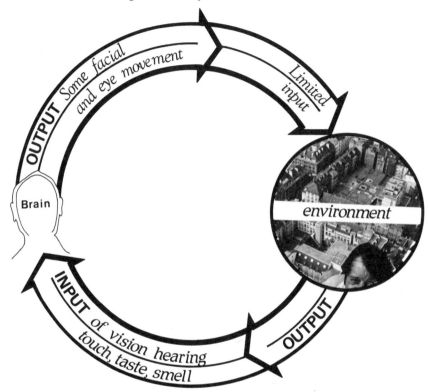

Fig. 8.1. Blockage on the output side of the loop

The four possible awareness states of the patient

The possible states of awareness of the patient are:

1. The Comatose and Unresponsive State

This means that there is no response to any stimulus in any way. There is no facial expression, no change in heart rate for breathing, and no movement of the limbs.

2. The Comatose But Responsive State

This means that when a stimulus is given to the senses of the patient, either by sight, hearing, touch, smell or taste, there will be a response. This response may be knowledge of how to deal with the problems which you have at present and also by increased breathing, increased heart rate, facial expression, or movement of a limb or the body.

3. The Conscious But Unresponsive State

If the patient has no way of responding or indicating to us correctly an awareness of our presence, then *we* tend to think that he or she has no brain working.

This may be totally inaccurate. The patient may be "locked in" and unable to obey a command (see Chapter 23). They may be able to pick up the sensations of seeing and hearing and feeling and even taste and smell, but unable to give us any indication that they can. They cannot provide a response to become our stimulus.

Even if the patient is capable of making some movement, it may not be the one that is requested from them. If they can only move their left leg, but are asked to move their right arm, then they may respond by moving their left leg, because that is the only movement which they can do. It is, therefore, very easy to think that the patient cannot provide you with a correct response to your request, and you may seriously misinterpret what they are attempting to show you.

4. The Conscious and Responsive State

In this state the patient is out of coma and can demonstrate this by obeying a simple command. In other words, if you ask him or her to move the hand towards your face, or lift up a leg, s/he can do it and repeat it. It is important to know that patients may be conscious and responsive in the morning, when they are fresh, but poorly responsive later in the day, when they are tired. They will also respond to different people in a different manner, and some patients may totally ignore people whom they do not like. Also if they are constipated or have a high temperature, they will often not respond or respond poorly.

This brings up a most important concept. The concept of the "Fragile Period".

The fragile period

Unfortunately the medical profession only wishes to know of "hard facts" (facts that can be repeated and verified by other people). This is all related to the so-called "scientific method" of gaining knowledge, the ability to measure, weigh and count everything.

It seems unbelievable that the profession has not yet understood that many of the most basic factors in life cannot be weighed, measured, counted, etc. Love, hope, faith, forgiveness, joy, beauty, etc., cannot be measured by the scientific method with any degree of accuracy.

This fragile period has so far not been measured, and it may not be able to be measured with the tools which we have at our disposal at present. It is the period between the points when the patient has an awareness, no matter how primitive, of the environment, and when that awareness can be demonstrated by the scientific method (that is, when the patient obeys a command). The early indications of awareness are dealt with in the following two chapters.

This fragile period may be of great importance as the patient arousing from coma, surrounded by a totally foreign and threatening environment and incapable of communicating properly either by voice or any other motor action, withdraws and closes down his mental processes.

In diagram form the fragile period is like this:

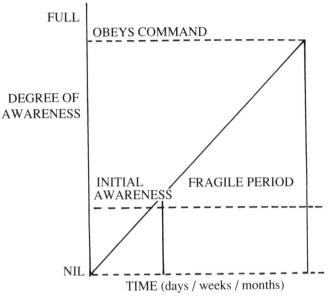

Fig. 8.2. The Fragile Period

Many relatives find that they can obtain a response during the fragile period when no one else can. They may also find that the response may be better with one relative than with others.

You have to decide whether the patient is:

1. COMATOSE AND UNRESPONSIVE.
2. COMATOSE AND RESPONSIVE.
3. CONSCIOUS AND UNRESPONSIVE.
4. CONSCIOUS AND RESPONSIVE.

IF THE PATIENT IS IN 2 OR 3, THEN IT IS VERY LIKELY THAT S/HE IS IN THE FRAGILE PERIOD, AND IT IS WISE FOR YOU TO BE VERY CONSIDERATE IN YOUR DEALINGS WITH HIM OR HER.

You have now to work out how much the patient is picking up from their world, even though they are apparently, or truly, in coma.

In my experience and that of my Coma Arousal nurses, and of many other nurses, the relatives know best how the patient is responding to the environment.

You need to pool this knowledge. All those who are closely concerned with the patient, and spend some time with him or her, need to sit down and discuss the questions and fill in the questionnaire in the next chapter.

Invite a member of the medical or nursing staff to sit in on the discussion.

Do not be swayed by the opinion of the doctor or nurse. Take note of it, for they are professionals. It is highly likely, however, that you are with the patient much more than they are and, as a result, more able to provide the information.

Have you the authority to assess the patient?

If you wish to provide a programme in an effort to arouse the patient from coma, it is very likely that you will be running against accepted medical opinion. To be able to do this, you must be able to detect the changes in the patient which the doctor and nurse may not be aware of.

To do this you must undertake an assessment of the patient. You will not have to do a medical examination of the patient. Most of what you need to know will be easily observed by you.

Do you have any authority to do this assessment? The answer is YES!

The medical officer has the authority from *status*, given by his knowledge and legal position, and the relative has authority from *function*, given by time and love and knowledge of the patient and also by a legal position.

The position of each of you, the medical officer and the relative, has been stated in another context by Richard Foster in his book, *Celebration of Discipline* (Hodder and Stoughton, 1980), when he talks about "the Authority of Function and not of Status".

You have the authority of function. By your love, concern, time, commitment, you have the right of this authority.

It is of great benefit if the two authorities can be combined to work together for the good of the patient. In all walks of life, though, the authority relating to status does not like to work with the authority relating to function, and may try and reject cooperation.

You have heard of "People Power". That is what you are, using it now for the sake of the patient. Do not abdicate your position of authority of function, once you have made your stand.

If you are not confident that the nurse or medical officer will be sensitive or responsive, then do not invite them to your initial meeting of relatives, friends, etc. If they are tending to "put you down", meet without them.

Have your first meeting, and then ask the medical officer to the next meeting, to explain the information that you have obtained from the questionnaire.

To be fair to the medical officer, you should provide a copy of your findings a few days before the meeting, so that he or she may have adequate time to look at what you have found.

DO NOT EXPECT THE MEDICAL OFFICER TO SEE THE SAME THINGS YOU SEE.
THEY DO NOT HAVE THE SAME AMOUNT OF TIME TO SPEND WITH THE PATIENT AS YOU DO.
THEY DO NOT KNOW THE PATIENT AS WELL AS YOU DO.
THEY CANNOT, THEREFORE, SEE OR KNOW AS MUCH.

If the medical officer does come to the meeting, then hold fast to your views. Do not be intimidated.

Before you start with the discussion and questionnaire, you should also understand a few other points.

1. The information which you pool will be "soft" information. In other words, it is often difficult to be certain of it.

2. Much of what you see, you will be unsure of. You may only get a fleeting impression. This should not be discounted, it should be noted with the words "not confirmed".

3. If something is confirmed, but is not seen all the time it should be noted as "present", but "variable".

4. You will often find that the patient is much better in responding at certain times of the ,day. This is usually in the morning, but may also vary, depending upon the amount of drug therapy being given.

5. Another major factor relates to problems with the bowels. If the patient is constipated, s/he may be very irritable or unresponsive. Repeatedly, I have seen patients who are very restless and very unresponsive improve dramatically after an enema.

6. In general, the patient should be out of bed and sitting up, in the upright position, as much as possible. If this cannot be done the head of the bed should be elevated. Sometimes patients must be bedridden because of damage to other parts of the body.
   (You must not change the position of the patient without the permission of the charge nurse in the ward.)

7. Understand that you will have differing opinions, because you will not all see the same things. Anything positive must be noted, even if you do write "not confirmed" or "variable".

8. Do not argue among yourselves as to what you see. It is unlikely that you will be asked to stand in the dock of a court of law and swear to anything which you see or say. Do not dispute among yourselves. Note what all say, for it is amazing how some person will see something even two weeks or more before anyone else.

So

A. Select a day when all those interested can be present.

B. Meet within the hospital or a place convenient to the majority of the group.

C. Select someone to read out the questions one at a time.

D. Spend as much time as you like on each question.

E. Have a second person, with a photostat of the questionnaire gather the information also and complete the form.

Any parts which you cannot answer, mark in "UNKNOWN".

It is also wise to read Chapter 10, "The Dawn of Awareness", before you come to the meeting so that you will be able to sit together and write down what your conclusions are.

When you have finished, type out a report, send a copy to the medical officer, and ask for an interview time to discuss the findings.

CHAPTER 9

THE QUESTIONNAIRE TO FIND OUT THE

STATE OF THE PATIENT

Introduction

It is extremely important that YOU, who are most involved with the patient, should fill in the questionnaire. No one is more qualified than you are. You will be more accurate than the hospital staff because you know the patient well and spend more time with him or her.

There are a few simple tests which you will have to do, but most of the information you or your family or friends will pick up is by observation of the patient.

The only equipment you will need will be a 9-volt torch, a nailbrush and a vibrator. The torch is to shine in the patient's eyes to see if the pupil reacts to light. If you have any difficulty with this, ask one of the medical or nursing staff for help. The nailbrush is to test the patient's reaction to pain. To test for this reaction, just press the back of the nail brush firmly against the thumbnail or the big-toenail and watch for the reaction. If you do not like doing this, then you may ask one of the doctors or nurses to do it. Otherwise you may obtain your answer by exerting pressure on the hair on the arm or leg. In all your testing there is no need to be hurtful, and if you have any doubts, ask for help from the staff.

As you fill in the questions, you must mark where you finish getting the positive answers. This will indicate the highest level the patient has reached at this stage. You must place that information in the chart at the end of this chapter by cross hatching the correct stage.

As the patient comes out of coma and recovers function, he or she will go through different stages. The levels of the Glasgow Coma Scale detailed in Chapter 2 is the basis for the stages. The easiest way to both chart and understand the recovery process is to think in terms of steps up which the patient climbs (see Chapter 15, "The Pathway of Recovery"). There are two sets of steps: one is Sensory and one is Motor, with five steps in each. We will call each step a STAGE.

The meaning of the questionnaire and the answers you obtain from it are dealt with in detail in the next three chapters. It would be wise for you to read these chapters before you fill in the questionnaire, and return to them for clarification of any points.

THE *SENSORY STAGES* are:

Stage 5	THE DISCRIMINATING STAGE
Stage 4	THE LOCALIZING STAGE
Stage 3	THE WITHDRAWAL STAGE
Stage 2	THE REFLEX STAGE
Stage 1	NO REACTION

THE *MOTOR STAGES* are:

Stage 5	FINE CONTROLLED MOVEMENT
Stage 4	CONTROLLED MOVEMENT
Stage 3	SPONTANEOUS MOVEMENT
Stage 2	REFLEX MOVEMENT
Stage 1	NO REACTION

The organisation of the Questionnaire

1   PROGNOSIS
2   VIGILANCE
3   EMOTION
4   DRIVE

SENSORY ASSESSMENTS

5   VISUAL FUNCTION
6   AUDITORY FUNCTION
7   TACTILE FUNCTION

MOTOR ASSESSMENTS

8   STAGE ONE — NO MOVEMENT
9   STAGE TWO — REFLEX MOVEMENT
10   STAGE THREE — SPONTANEOUS MOVEMENT
11   STAGE FOUR — CONTROLLED MOVEMENT
12   STAGE FIVE — FINE CONTROLLED MOVEMENT
13   HAND FUNCTION
14   VOCALIZATION
15   SWALLOWING

The following are the questions which you need to answer.
If you find any questions which do not fit the patient, move on to the next question.
If you do not have the information, write UNKNOWN.

YES | NO

1   *PROGNOSIS*

1.1   What have you been told about the *condition* of the patient? S/He has been:
 1.1.1   Moderately brain injured.
 1.1.2   Severely brain injured.

1.2   What have you been told about the *prognosis* of the patient? The chances are that s/he will:
 1.2.1   Make a good recovery.
 1.2.2   Be moderately disabled.
 1.2.3   Be severely disabled.
 1.2.4   Be vegetative.
 1.2.5   Probably die.

2   *VIGILANCE*

2.1   Do you think that the patient knows if you, or others, are present in any way?

2.2   Does the patient react differently depending upon who is present?

2.3   Does the patient react differently when the environment is changed?

2.4
 2.4.1   Does the patient open his/her eyes?
 2.4.2   Is the extent of eye-opening full?
 2.4.3   Is the extent of eye-opening limited?
 2.4.4   Does only the right eye open?
 2.4.5   Does only the left eye open?
 2.4.6   Is the speed of opening normal?
 2.4.7   Is the speed of opening slow?
 2.4.8   Is the duration of eye-opening long? (hours)
 2.4.9   Is the duration of eye-opening moderate? (minutes)
 2.4.10   Is the duration of eye-opening short? (seconds)

2.5

    2.5.1   Is this eye-opening spontaneous, that is, occurs without you doing anything to the patient?

    2.5.2   Is this eye-opening in response to voice?

    2.5.3   Is this eye-opening in response to pain ?

2.6

    2.6.1   How many hours does the patient appear to sleep in the day ?

                                day . . . hours,

    2.6.2   How many hours does the patient appear to sleep in the night?

                               night . . . hours.

---

3   *EMOTION*

3.1   Are there facial changes of

    3.1.1   anxiety?

    3.1.2   fear?

    3.1.3   anger?

    3.1.4   sadness?

    3.1.5   any tears?

    3.1.6   disgust?

    3.1.7   contempt?

    3.1.8   surprise?

    3.1.9   pleasure?

3.2

    3.2.1   Is there movement of the eyebrows?

    3.2.2   Is there movement of the nose?

    3.2.3   Is there movement of the the lips?

---

4   *DRIVE*

Is there any evidence of independence?

4.1   Does the patient resist some of the things which you do to him/her?

Example 1

Example 2

4.2   Does the patient co-operate with some of the things which you do to him/her?

    Example 1

    Example 2

Sensory assessments

5   *VISUAL FUNCTION*

5.1   If the eyes do not move, what position are the eyes?
    5.1.1   Do they look to the right?
    5.1.2   Do they look to the left?
    5.1.3   Does one look to the right and one to the left?
    5.1.4   Are they in the midline?

5.2
    5.2.1   Are both pupils the same size?
    5.2.2   Is the right pupil larger?
    5.2.3   Is the left pupil larger?

STAGE 1   NO REACTION STAGE

    If the pupils do not change in size when you shine the torch (see question 5.3) mark STAGE 1 in Chart 1 at the end of the chapter.

STAGE 2   REFLEX STAGE

5.3
    5.3.1   When you shine a 9-volt torch into the eyes does the right pupil stay the same?
    5.3.2   When you shine a 9-volt torch into the eyes does the right pupil become smaller?
    5.3.3   When you shine a 9-volt torch into the eyes does the left pupil stay the same?
    5.3.4   When you shine a 9-volt torch into the eyes does the left pupil become smaller?

    If the pupils change in size when you shine the torch, then mark STAGE 2 in Chart 1 at the end of the chapter.

STAGE 3   WITHDRAWAL STAGE

5.4

5.4.1   When you touch the eyelid gently with your finger, does the right eyelid blink or move?
5.4.2   When you touch the eyelid gently with your finger, does the left eyelid blink or move?

5.5

5.5.1   When you shine the torch into the right eye, does the right eyelid blink or move?
5.5.2   When you shine the torch into the left eye, does the left eyelid blink or move?

5.6

5.6.1   When you move your fingers towards the right eye without touching the eyelid, does the right eyelid blink or move?
5.6.2   When you move your fingers towards the left eye without touching the eyelid, does the left eyelid blink or move?

If the eyelids blink when you shine the torch, then mark STAGE 3 in Chart 1 at the end of the chapter.

STAGE 4   LOCALIZING STAGE

5.7

5.7.1   Is there scanning, that is, does the right eye move around even when there is no visual stimulus?
5.7.2   Is there scanning, that is, does the left eye move around like a radar even when there is no visual stimulus?

5.8   Do the eyes move together, i.e, in unison?

5.9   Is there any movement of the eyes or head towards a visual stimulus?

5.10

5.10.1   Do you think that the right eye looks at a light?
5.10.2   Do you think that the left eye looks at a light?
5.10.3   Do you think that the right eye looks at an object?
5.10.4   Do you think that the left eye looks at an object?

5.10.5	Do you think that the right eye looks at a face?
5.10.6	Do you think that the left eye looks at a face?

5.11

5.11.1	Does the right eye follow a light?
5.11.2	Does the left eye follow a light?
5.11.3	Does the right eye follow an object?
5.11.4	Does the left eye follow an object?
5.11.5	Does the right eye follow a face?
5.11.6	Does the left eye follow a face?

If an eye looks at or follows a visual stimulus, mark STAGE 4 in Chart 1 at the end of the chapter.

STAGE 5   DISCRIMINATING STAGE

5.12

5.12.1	Do you think there is any eye contact between you and the patient with the right eye?
5.12.2	Do you think there is any eye contact between you and the patient with the left eye?

If an eye makes eye contact, then mark STAGE 5 in Chart 1 at the end of the chapter.

5.13

5.13.1	Does the patient appear to recognize photographs?
5.13.2	Does the patient appear to recognize pictures?
5.13.3	Does the patient appear to recognize people? (without talking to the patient)

6   *AUDITORY FUNCTION*

STAGE 1   NO REACTION
If the answer to question 6.1 is NO, then mark STAGE 1 in Chart 1 at the end of chapter.

STAGE 2   REFLEX STAGE

6.1   Does the patient blink or move if you make a loud noise
(e.g, with a klaxon horn or loud whistle)?
If the answer is YES, mark STAGE 2 in Chart 1 at the end
of the chapter.

STAGE 3   WITHDRAWAL STAGE

6.2   If you continue the noise, does the patient stop blinking or
moving?

If the answer is YES, mark STAGE 3 in Chart 1 at the end
of the chapter.

STAGE 4   LOCALIZING STAGE

6.3

6.3.1   Does the patient turn the eyes towards the noise?
6.3.2   Does the patient turn the head towards the noise?

If the answer is YES to either, mark STAGE 4 in Chart 1 at
the end of the chapter.

STAGE 5   DISCRIMINATING STAGE

6.4   Does the patient appear to recognize a known voice?

6.5   Does the patient appear to recognise the tone of the voice?

6.6   Will the patient relax if asked to do so?

6.7   Does the patient respond to words in an appropriate
manner?

6.8   Has the patient obeyed a command?

If the answer is YES to 6.7 or 6.8, mark STAGE 5 in Chart
1 at end of chapter.

7 *TACTILE FUNCTION* GENERAL QUESTIONS

7.1 Does the patient appear to feel pain?
7.2
    7.2.1 Does the patient appear to feel heat or cold?
    7.2.2 Does the patient relax in the bath?
7.3 Does the patient become more aware (e.g, eye-open, grimace) when touched?

7.4 Does the patient appear to register discomfort?

7.5 Does the patient react in any way when his/her body or limbs are moved?

STAGE 1 NO REACTION

If the answer to 7.5 or 7.6 or 7.7 is NO then mark STAGE 1 in Chart 1 at the end of the chapter.

STAGE 2 REFLEX STAGE

7.6
    7.6.1 Does the patient *stretch* the arms when you apply pain?
    7.6.2 Does the patient *stretch* the legs when you apply pain?

7.7
    7.7.1 Does the patient *bend* the arms when you apply pain?
    7.7.1 Does the patient *bend* the legs when you apply pain?

If the answer is YES, then mark STAGE 2 in Chart 1.

STAGE 3 WITHDRAWAL STAGE

7.8
    7.8.1 If you apply pain to the right arm does the patient only move *that* arm?
    7.8.2 If you apply pain to the left arm does the patient only move *that* arm?

91

7.8.3   If you apply pain to the right leg does the patient only move *that* leg?

7.8.4   If you apply pain to the left leg does the patient only move *that* leg?

If the answer is YES then mark STAGE 3 in Chart 1 at the end of the chapter.

STAGE 4   LOCALIZING STAGE

7.9

7.9.1   If you squeeze the ear, does the patient move the hand in the direction of the ear?

7.9.2   If you apply pain to an arm or leg, does the patient move the other arm or leg so as to push away the cause of the pain?

7.10

7.10.1   If you apply ice to the abdomen, does the patient move the arm to push away the ice?

If the answer is YES then mark STAGE 4. on Chart 1 at the end of the chapter.

STAGE 5   DISCRIMINATING STAGE

7.11

7.11.1   Can the patient indicate to you by touching an object whether it is hot?

7.11.2   Can the patient indicate to you by touching an object whether it is cold?

7.11.3   Can the patient indicate to you by touching an object whether it is hard?

7.11.4   Can the patient indicate to you by touching an object whether it is soft?

7.11.5   Can the patient indicate to you by touching an object whether it is rough?

7.11.6   Can the patient indicate to you by touching an object whether it is smooth?

If the answer is YES to any of these questions, mark STAGE 5 on Chart 1 at the end of the chapter.

Motor assessments

8   STAGE 1   NO MOVEMENT

8.1   Does the patient reflexly move any part of his/her body or limbs? Reflexly, meaning if you make a noise or touch the patient, the patient will move.

If the answer is NO, mark STAGE 1 in Chart 2 (Limb and Body Movement) at the end of the chapter.

8.2   If the patient does not move, what is his/her position?
8.2.1   Arms bent at elbows / legs bent at knees?
8.2.2   Arms bent at elbows / legs straight at knees?
8.2.3   Arms straight at elbows / legs bent at knees?
8.2.4   Arms straight at elbows / legs straight at knees?

9   STAGE 2   REFLEX MOVEMENT

9.1   Are there any reflex movements? Reflex, meaning if you make a noise, use a light, or touch the patient, the patient will move.

If the answer is YES, then mark STAGE 2 in Chart 2 at the end of the chapter.

9.1.1   Is the reflex movement a total body movement? (i.e, marked 2 or 3 on the Motor Section, Glasgow Coma Scale).
9.1.2   How strong are the total body reflex movements?
1   Strong?
2   Moderate?
3   Weak?
9.1.3   How long do the total body movements last?
1   Short (i.e, less than 30 secs)?
2   Moderate (30 secs to 2 mins)?
3   Long (over 2 mins)?
9.1.4   How frequent are the total body movements?
1   Very frequent?
2   Frequent?
3   Rare?
9.1.5   What brings them on?
1   Noise?
2   Touch?

93

    3   Light?

    4   Movement?

9.1.6   Can you stop the movements by talking to the patient?

9.1.7   Can you stop the movements by touching the patient?

9.2   Is the reflex a local withdrawal?

---

10   STAGE 3   SPONTANEOUS MOVEMENTS

Spontaneous movements are movements which occur without you apparently doing anything to the patient.

If the answer to any of questions 10.1 — 10.6 is YES, then mark STAGE 3.

10.1   Are there any spontaneous movements of the head?
    10.1.1   Turns to either side?
    10.1.2   Lifts up head from the chest?

10.2   Are there any spontaneous movements of the body?
    10.2.1   Does the patient wriggle or change his/her position?

10.3   Are there any spontaneous movements of the right arm? With his/her right hand: does s/he touch:
    10.3.1   the head?
    10.3.2   the face?
    10.3.3   the chest?
    10.3.4   the abdomen?
    10.3.5   the groin?
    10.3.6   the thigh?
    10.3.7   the other hand?

Does s/he stretch out the right arm:
    10.3.8   in front?
    10.3.9   to the side?
    10.3.10   to the back?

10.4   Are there any spontaneous movements of the left arm? With the left hand: does s/he touch:
    10.4.1   the head?
    10.4.2   the face?
    10.4.3   the chest?
    10.4.4   the abdomen?

10.4.5   the groin?
10.4.6   the thigh?
10.4.7   the other hand?

Does s/he stretch out the left arm:
10.4.8   in front?
10.4.9   to the side?
10.4.10   to the back?

10.5   Are there any spontaneous movements of the right leg?
    10.5.1   Does s/he stretch it out?
    10.5.2   Does s/he bend it?

    Are there any spontaneous movements of the left leg?
    10.5.3   Does s/he stretch it out?
    10.5.4   Does s/he bend it?

10.6   Is there any tremor(shaking)?

---

11   STAGE 4   CONTROLLED MOVEMENT

Controlled movements we will define as "movements in response to a command or request."

If the answer to any of questions 11.1 — 11.6 is YES, mark STAGE 4 in Chart 2 at the end of the chapter.

11.1   Will s/he obey a request to move the head?
    11.1.1   Turns to either side?
    11.1.2   Lifts up head from the chest?

11.2   Does the patient wriggle or change his/her position if asked to do so?

11.3   Are there any controlled movements of the right arm?
    With the right hand does s/he touch:
    11.3.1   the head?
    11.3.2   the face?
    11.3.3   the chest?
    11.3.4   the abdomen?
    11.3.5   the groin?
    11.3.6   the thigh?
    11.3.7   the other hand?

Does s/he stretch out the right arm:
11.3.8   in front?
11.3.9   to the side?
11.3.10   to the back?

11.4   Are there any controlled movements of the left arm? With the left hand: does s/he touch:
11.4.1   the head?
11.4.2   the face?
11.4.3   the chest?
11.4.4   the abdomen?
11.4.5   the groin?
11.4.6   the thigh?
11.4.7   the other hand?

Does s/he stretch out the left arm:
11.4.8   in front?
11.4.9   to the side?
11.4.10   to the back?

11.5   Are there any controlled movements of the right leg?
11.5.1   Does s/he stretch it out?
11.5.2   Does s/he bend it?

Are there any controlled movements of the left leg?
11.5.3   Does s/he stretch it out?
11.5.4   Does s/he bend it?

12   STAGE 5   FINE CONTROLLED MOVEMENT

If the patient can perform fine controlled movements in correct sequence, then s/he is well out of coma and has regained a significant level of function. You should mark STAGE 5 on Chart 2 at the end of the chapter.

13   *HAND FUNCTION*

STAGE 1   NO MOVEMENT

13.1

13.1.1   Is there any movement of the right hand?
13.1.2   Is there any movement of the left hand?
If the answer to question 13.1 is NO, mark STAGE 1 in Chart 2 (Hand Function)at the end of the chapter.

STAGE 2   REFLEX MOVEMENT

13.2

    13.2.1   Does his/her right hand hold yours when you place your hand in his/her palm?
    13.2.2   Does his/her left hand hold yours when you place your hand in his/her palm?

If the answer is YES, mark STAGE 2 in Chart 2 at the end of the chapter.

STAGE 3   SPONTANEOUS MOVEMENT

13.3

    13.3.1   Does the index finger on the right hand point?
    13.3.2   Does the index finger on the left hand point?
    13.3.3   Do the fingers on the right hand open?
    13.3.4   Do the fingers on the left hand open?
If the answer to any questions in 13.3 is YES, mark STAGE 3 in Chart 2. at the end of the chapter.

STAGE 4   CONTROLLED MOVEMENT

13.4

    13.4.1   Can s/he take something in the right palm and hold it when you ask him/her?
    13.4.2   Can s/he take something in the left palm and hold it when you ask him/her?
    13.4.3   Can s/he release the grasp on an object with the right hand when you request?
    13.4.4   Can s/he release the grasp on an object with the left hand when you request?

If the answer to any questions in 13.4 is YES, mark STAGE 4 in Chart 2. at the end of the chapter.

STAGE 5   FINE CONTROLLED MOVEMENT

13.5

    13.5.1   Can s/he hold something between the finger and thumb in the right hand?
    13.5.2   Can s/he hold something between the finger and thumb in the left hand?

If the answer is YES to any of 13.5 mark STAGE 5 in the Chart at the end of the chapter.

14   *VOCALIZATION*

While it is unlikely that the patient will make a sound while the tracheostomy is in place, it can occur.
If there is no sound, mark STAGE 1 in the section marked Vocalization in Chart 2 at end of chapter.

14.1 Does s/he make any sound?
       If there is any sound, mark STAGE 2 in Chart 2 at end of chapter.
14.2 Does s/he say any words?
       If any words are used mark STAGE 3 in Chart 2 at end of chapter.

14.3 Does s/he join any words together, even if they appear confused?
       If any words are joined together mark STAGE 4 in Chart 2 at end of chapter.

14.4 Does s/he have conversation which is correct?

       If correct conversation occurs mark STAGE 5 in Chart 2 at end of chapter.

15   *SWALLOWING*

15.1 Is there much saliva?
15.2 Can s/he swallow?

15.3 Does s/he cough?

These charts will allow you to determine where the patient is as far as conscious state and function are concerned. Select from your questionnaire the correct Stage for each function and *crosshatch it on to* the chart.
Always check twice and crosshatch once.

Questions 1.1 to 7.11.6

	Visual	*Auditory*	*Tactile*
STAGE 1	No response	No response	No response
STAGE 2	Pupillary response	Startle reflex	Extension flexion response
STAGE 3	Blink to touch, light, confrontation	Habituation	Withdrawal of limb
STAGE 4	Localizes visual stimuli	Localizes auditory stimuli	Localizes tactile stimuli
STAGE 5	Eye contact Visual recognition	Comprehends auditory input	Discriminates tactile input

CHART 2

MOTOR FUNCTIONS

Questions 8.1 to 14.4

	Limb and Body Movement	Hand Function	Vocalization
STAGE 1	No movement	No movement	No sound
STAGE 2	Reflex movement	Grasp reflex	Sounds
STAGE 3	Spontaneous movement	E.T. sign Hand release	Use of words
STAGE 4	Control of movement	Prehensile grasp	Use of sentences
STAGE 5	Fine control of movement	Pincer grasp	Correct conversation

In Chapter 8 the four possible states are listed. These are:

1 The Comatose and Unresponsive State

If NO REACTION is listed for all functions, then the patient is in this category. This is extremely unusual, except in the early stages of coma.

2 The Comatose but Responsive State

Most patients will show some evidence of response, and the majority of patients will be in this category, the details of which are expanded in the next three chapters.

3 The Conscious but Unresponsive State

This is what is regarded as the "locked in" state. See Chapter 23. If you feel the patient is conscious, but is not responding, go back and do the questionnaire again.

4. The Conscious and Responsive State

This is the state which is being aimed for. Even when this is accomplished there is still a great deal of work to be done to restore good function to the patient.

This questionnaire is the basis for all your work as you seek to arouse the patient from coma. It is also a tool which you can use to see the progress which you may make with the patient.

BE SURE THAT YOU KEEP ALL RECORDS IN A SAFE PLACE.

DUPLICATE ALL RECORDS SO THAT IN THE EVENT OF LOSS, THERE IS ALWAYS ONE AVAILABLE.

CHAPTER 10

THE DAWN OF AWARENESS

Introductory Statement

Professor Charles Tart, professor of psychology at the University of California, Davis, states:

> We begin with a concept of some kind of basic awareness, some kind of basic ability to 'know' or 'sense' or 'recognize' that something is happening. This is a fundamental theoretical and experiential given. We do not know scientifically what the nature of awareness is, but it is our starting point.

> Tart, C.T. *Altered States of Consciousness.*
> (New York: Macmillan, 1977)

Professor Tart talks our language. The starting point of our quest in the brain injured patient is to find out if there is any awareness of the environment. We cannot, at this time, tell scientifically what this starting point is; but we would agree that it is a concept of some kind of basic awareness, of an ability to recognize that something is happening.

This chapter will work with questions 1 to 4, relating to the prognosis, vigilance/awareness, the emotional output and the drive of the patient, and explain what they mean.

Your Attitude

Do you still see the patient as a person? Many who deal with such patients will not see them as persons. They will consider that they have no brain functioning and are vegetable-like creatures, and that is how they will be treated unless you can establish that they are not vegetables and are still people. To do this takes time and patience and documentation.

You may be up against the caring professions when you start now to note closely how the patient is responding and to interpret your information. You must be careful and cautious and stick very closely to what you see and feel.

For all practical purposes what you will be undertaking is, firstly, to get the patient out of coma and, secondly, to attempt to restore function to the patient. To put it another way, you must wake the patient up and then help him or her back toward a normal life. Until the patient is awake, a start on the path to recovery cannot be made. There are, therefore, two parts to this work.

PART ONE — TO WAKE THE PATIENT UP

PART TWO — TO RESTORE THE FUNCTION OF THE PATIENT

The questionnaire you have filled in will be the basis of all the work you will do. Before you start, however, you need to know: Is there any response from the patient and what is it? The sections of the questionnaire which will provide some information on whether the patient is capable of being aroused are concerned with Vigilance, Eye-opening, Emotional response, and Drive or Independence. Each of these will be dealt with in turn followed by information on what the responses mean as far as Vision, Hearing, Touch and Movement are concerned.

1 PROGNOSIS

Question 1.
What have you been told about the condition of the patient?

You may have been told different things by different doctors, all of which could have been right at the time. If this has occurred, then whoever can communicate best with the most senior doctor involved with the patient should make contact and ask for a clear statement about the position of the patient and what is likely to happen in the immediate future.

Question 1.2
What have you been told about the prognosis of the patient?

Have you been told that the patient will

1.2.1	make a good recovery.
1.2.2	make a moderate recovery.
1.2.3	be severely disabled.
1.2.4	be vegetative.
1.2.5	probably die.

(Do not forget to note who told you and when.) What do these terms mean?

The following is based on the Glasgow Outcome Scale.

1.2.1 *Good recovery* does not necessarily imply that the patient will recover and be able to function in the same way as before the accident. It means that the patient will be able to look after herself or himself, will be able to use transport, either personal or public, and may even be able to do some work. Just as you will be a different person after you have lived through this ordeal, it is reasonable to assume that the patient will be also.

1.2.2 *Moderate recovery* implies that the patient is able to look after himself or herself, if necessary in a hostel. He or she may need some help for certain activities, but is really seen as being independent for personal activities.

1.2.3 *Severely disabled* means that the patient is dependent upon other people for help and support for the majority of activities. It usually means hospitalization or living in an institution for total care.

1.2.4 In the *persistent vegetative state* the patient is considered to be mindless and incapable of meaningful contact with other persons. The term "vegetable" is frequently used, which is regrettable, and work which is currently being done indicates that the number of patients with this diagnosis may be much less than has been previously thought.

2 VIGILANCE

Question 2.1
Do you think the patient knows if you, or others, are present in any way?

This really means: How awake is the patient or aware of people? It is a measure of brainstem function.

If there is no response by the patient to people, or to changes in his or her environment, then the patient is deeply in coma (i.e., unresponsive).

Question 2.2
Does the patient react differently depending upon who is present?

Often we have found that patients will react more to a member of the family with whom there has been a very close relationship. Often they will react differently to their mother/father/sister/brother/wife /husband/friend. Often if you ask the nursing staff, they will tell you that one nurse can get a better response from the patient than the others.

Question 2.3
Does the patient react differently when the environment is changed?

If there is no obvious change in the reaction of the patient to different people (which in my experience, except in the early stages, is unlikely), then they may react to a change in their environment. Is there any change if the patient is shifted to another ward? Perhaps, in the move to the X-ray or another department or a new ward, there has been a reaction.

There is sometimes a reaction when the sucker is switched on to suck out the tracheostomy tube. The same may occur when the floor polisher is turned on by the ward cleaner. The sound may be similar to the sucker.

If the patient has done any of these things, reacted to different people or to a different situation in his or her environment, then he or she has some relationship with that environment (i.e., there may be an awareness of the environment and the patient must be treated as a person).

Question 2.4
Relating to eye-opening

Eye-opening is very important. It is a very primitive function. You can't use your sight if you don't have your eyes open. It is a prerequisite of vision.

It is very likely that within the first few days or even up to two weeks both eyes will be closed. It is always a good sign when the eyes start to open. Many people think that this means the patient is out of coma, but this is not necessarily true. The patient is not necessarily out of coma when the eyes open.

Nevertheless, it is still an important move forward. Sometimes, only one eye will open and the other will not open, or open only partially. This often means that the nerve supplying that eyelid has been damaged. (Sometimes the eyes won't open, because they are swollen, especially if there is damage around the eyelids or on the forehead.)

Obviously, it is better if eye-opening occurs at a normal speed, but this may take time to develop, especially if there has been damage to the nerve controlling this movement.

You will also find that initially the eyes may only be open for a few minutes, but usually as the days pass, they stay open longer.

Question 2.5.1
Is this eye-opening spontaneous?

If the eyes of the patient appear to be open many times when you enter the room and there is no one else present, it is reasonable to assume that spontaneous eye opening is occurring. This is a good thing.

Questions 2.5.2 and 2.5.3
Is eye-opening in response to voice or pain?

At first the eyes may only open when something painful is done to the patient. Then they may open if the patient is moved or shaken. Then they may open to a noise or to a voice.

In general, the more the eyes are open, the better. You can't take in anything of your environment visually without eye-opening, and vision is a very important part of the way in which we judge our environment.

Questions 2.6.1 and 2.6.2
Does the patient appear to sleep?

While patients are in coma, they appear to be asleep all the time. As they come out of coma, a sleep/wake pattern will often occur. This means that the patient appears to be awake for certain parts of the day, but will sleep at night.

3   EMOTION

Questions 3.1.1 to 3.1.9
Are there facial changes of emotion?

There are many ways in which we show emotion. If you refer back to Chapter 5, you will note that "hot brain" function is tied up with emotion. You are probably not an expert at identifying and measuring emotional outpouring in yourself, let alone in other people. We all know, however, to look at the face of a person to see how that person is feeling, because one way in which we all show emotion is through facial expression. It is very accurate and commences when we are a baby. It is body language and is very truthful.

Facial changes are very important to us. We are always on the lookout for them every time we see another person. It is part of the way in which we work our "approach distance". If someone gives you an "angry" look, you do not need to be told how the person feels. It is the same with a happy look. You do not need to be told how the person feels. It is obvious. Even in ordinary life no one likes to deal with someone who has a "poker" face. We all like to see the facial expression of those with whom we are dealing.

Even with the patient in coma or severely brain-injured we like to see facial expression. There are certain facial expressions which are basic and those are the ones listed in the questionnaire. They are anxiety, fear, anger, surprise, disgust, contempt, sadness and pleasure.

Even if they worry you, it is better for the patient to have facial expressions. As the patient comes out of coma, the family will often remark that the facial expressions are becoming more like the ones which the patient normally had. This must be seen as a good sign. Because of your relationship with the patient, you are probably more able to recognise an expression than anyone else and also identify what it means.

The most likely expressions to occur first are anxiety, fear or anger. Then you may have disgust or sadness, then at some future stage the patient may smile. This smiling may occur when you are talking and laughing with the patient, or when you make a joke of something that happened in the past and with which the patient is very familiar. Other signs of pleasure often come when the patient is having the hair brushed or stroked.

Sometimes the expressions come at special times, as when the physiotherapists are giving chest physiotherapy, or when some painful stimulus is given to the patient. A further step is when the patient starts to cry with the production of tears. This sometimes happens when you tell the patient that you are leaving. When this happens repeatedly, then you must be thinking, "How much does this person understand?"

The other interesting thing is that the face of the patient may start to return to normal as s/he improves, and relatives will often say, "S/He is beginning to look the same as before the accident." This may take months to occur in someone who is very severely brain-injured. In a manner of speaking, the face is the "barometer" of the patient's progress. It is almost as if the muscles of the face slowly regain their power, and what is known as their tone, which is really their tightness, as the patient improves.

Facial expression is dependent upon the nerve to the muscles of the face being able to work properly. There is a separate nerve to each side of the face that serves all the muscles on the one side. If one of these nerves has been damaged, it is very likely that the angle of the mouth will droop and saliva will dribble from that side. Recovery of this nerve tends to be very slow and prolonged and may not occur.

Questions 3.2.1 to 3.2.3
Is there movement of the eyebrows, nose, lips?

These questions are only to explore and provide information on the facial changes in slightly more detail.

4 INDEPENDENCE or DRIVE

Question 4.
Is there any evidence of independence (drive)?

One of the most important factors in life is the ability of the individual to be independent. We are, of course, all governed in what we do by circumstances, and while we strive for independence of thought and action, no one is a totally free agent.

The patient in coma often appears to have no independent actions, and we assume, because we cannot see any movement there is no independence of thought. This may not be the case. Often the reason we decide that there is no thinking brain is because we do not take enough notice of the small things which the patient does. We are used to seeing people make large movements and do big actions. It is obvious that the patient in coma is not able to move in a normal manner. We have to scale down our thinking and look for small actions and movements. Because we are not used to looking for such things, we often doubt that they are there. As you become more adept at looking and feeling, you will be more accurate in deciding what you are seeing.

Again, if we use normal living as our yardstick, it is obvious that when another person asks us to do something, if we are independent, we may either resist or we may co-operate. The choice is ours and we can demonstrate our independence.

With the patient in coma there may still be some evidence of independence. We must look closely for it, since it is of paramount importance to the patient's recovery that he or she should be able to come back to an independent state of thinking and action. Ask yourself: Does the patient indicate, in any way, their dislike of something being done to them and attempt to resist it?

Question 4.1
Does the patient resist some of the things you do to him/her?

One of the most likely things to occur is that the patient will make it difficult for you or the nurse to clean the teeth and will clench against the brush. This will often be a reflex action, but a reflex action is better than no action at all.

Other things of importance occur. You may have the feeling that the patient is resisting your movement of their arms or legs when you are giving a passive range of movement. Because many of these patients have increased tone or tightness in their muscles from the brain injury, it can be difficult to know if resistance is there or not. If over time, however, you note a change in the resistance, then it may be significant.

Question 4.2
Does the patient co-operate with some of the things you do to him/her?

Sometimes you may get the "feel" that the patient is helping you. Some people have noticed that when they are about to move a limb, or are moving a limb, or as they tell the patient what they are doing, the patient will give the impression of co-operating with them in the movement. In the early stages it is very difficult to be sure of this, but you should always keep your mind alive to it.

AGGRESSION

A separate note needs to be made on aggression or anger. As the patient comes out of coma, evidence of independence becomes more easily seen. Patients may resist quite forcefully when something is being done to them. They may become irritable and be regarded as difficult and aggressive. This is all perfectly normal.

As the patient's awareness of the environment increases, so does the realization that s/he is functioning below the normal level. If every time s/he tries to move an arm or a leg to do a specific action and fails miserably, or if when s/he attempts to speak, no words come or they hear some garbled sound which is not what they intended to say at all, then they become frustrated. If their performance is not up to the standard they expected, then frustration is inevitable. When frustration occurs, then hot brain takes over and anger follows. If poor ability to perform continues, and in the brain-injured patient this is inevitable for a long period of time, then the frustration continues and so does the anger. Anger which cannot be satisfied leads to aggression.

If we, in honesty, look at what happens to us when our performance is below what we hold as acceptable, we see the same pattern: poor performance — frustration — anger — aggression. The way we can deal with the problem is either to raise our performance or reduce the expectation we have of that performance. Both of these measures need to have cold brain functioning.

With patients who are brain-injured, there is no rapid way to improve performance. The only method open to them is to reduce expectation temporarily. They will have trouble understanding why this should be and will need constant reassurance that they will improve.

Aggression, then, is a constant factor which is positive and which, if channelled into a productive form, will lead to improved performance. To remove this anger by the use of drugs, except under exceptional circumstances and for short periods of time, is to reduce patients back to a level where even the poor function that they might have is taken away from them. To see brain-injured patients who are trying to express their frustration and anger, and seeking to regain function, drugged back into a comatose existence is very distressing.

Equally disastrous is to see the patient who has some spontaneous movement in an arm or leg, and is trying to use the limb, seeking to improve that movement, only to have it tied to the edge of the bed or to a bedrail. The patient who is wriggling his or her body, and wriggles out of the chair, is also demonstrating the need to try and regain independence. For them, to be tied around the waist to the back of a chair by a sheet, and to have another around their knees tying them to the legs or base of the chair, does not help them solve their problem; it compounds it.

These problems and what to do about them have already been discussed in detail in Chapter 7. It is important that you go back and read it.

CHAPTER 11

ASSESSING THE RETURN OF SENSATION

We are dealing here with the return of sensation, and with questions 5.1 to 7.11.6 which seek to show how the sensations of vision, hearing and touch gradually return in a hierarchical or developmental manner. We need to discuss the response of the patient to the environment in terms of vision, hearing and touch. These responses will allow us to know if the patient is taking in or processing any information by sensory pathways, and the level of function that has been obtained.

The easiest way to understand the return of function is to realize that every act we perform is sequential. If we are building a brick wall, we do so with one brick at a time, always starting with the bottom bricks. If we climb a ladder, we do so a step at a time, and we normally never start half-way up or at the top, but always at the bottom. If we start a journey, it is a step at a time, and we always start at the first step, never the last. If we learn to play the piano, a start is always made by the use of one note to which others are added; for a period of weeks or months, etc., simple tunes are played, but the direction is constantly towards a more complex or complicated piece of music.

It is the same with the way the brain processes information. The injured brain deals first in a simple way with the information given to it, and develops more complicated methods of dealing with the information as its function improves. There is always a sequence which the brain follows. Some people think this sequence or pattern is almost inflexible.

If the bricks in a wall are placed haphazardly, it will not function as a wall should. With music, there is always a sequence in which a piece is played. If this sequence is not followed, you are playing a different piece of music or merely producing noise.

In everything we do, we must commence at the right place and we must progress through the right sequence. There is always a pattern which must be followed.

Now, what I am saying is that the person who is brain-injured may not have all the thinking part of the brain working. If there is any response to the environment in the early stages, it is likely to be from the most primitive part of the brain (the brainstem). This is like laying the first bricks again. It is very early in brain function. It is in the brainstem that the mechanism for keeping us awake is most fully developed.

It is only when there is some awareness of the environment that the brain can take in and process information.

The process that you are hoping will occur is for the patient to establish function in their brainstem, and from that point start to establish more function in the rest of their brain.

This recovery of SENSORY function takes the five stages listed in Chapter 9. These stages are, commencing at the most primitive level:

1. No Reaction
2. Reflex Stage
3. Withdrawal Stage
4. Localizing Stage
5. Discriminating Stage
    a. Coarse discrimination
    b. Fine discrimination

I will go through each of these stages with vision, hearing and touch.

---

5   VISUAL FUNCTION

The easy way to understand visual function is to think of radar equipment. You have seen the way in which the sweeper moves around the radar screen and identifies any change in the pattern on the screen. Our eyes are very much like that sweeper. We move them constantly, depending upon the stimuli in our environment, in an effort to pick up any change. Any change picked up by our eyes may mean that we are in possible danger and must take avoiding action. In the brain-injured patient this ability to scan or sweep is often lost. It is essential to have this scanning ability, so that we may localize the position of stimuli in our environment and then identify it.

If we take this example and reduce it to its component parts we see that;

Firstly, the radar needs to be switched on, as the brain needs to be switched on by having awareness.

Secondly, the cover must be taken off the radar screen, as the eyelids need to be open.

Thirdly, the radar needs to have a scanning device, which can move through the environment, as the eyes need to rove around the environment.

Fourthly, the radar needs to fix, and if necessary pursue, a stimulus in the environment, as our eyes need to fix or localize on to and, if necessary, pursue an object.

Fifthly, the radar is only a tool to be used to determine where and what the stimulus is in a very coarse process of discrimination. It needs to be interpreted by the radar experts. In the same way our eyes need to identify the features of an object at which we look. It is the brain, however, that processes the information and decides what it is and what it means to the observer.

Our vision, therefore, depends basically upon three different components. These are *eyelid opening*, *eye movement* and *sight*. A deficiency in any one of these will

111

reduce the visual ability of the person. It is almost as if these three components occur in a sequence, with eye-opening being followed by movement of the eye towards the object, followed by the eye then focusing on the object, and transmitting the information to the brain.

Eye-opening has already been dealt with. After the eyelid is opened, the eye must be able to move if full function is to be obtained. Questions 5.1 to 5.13.3 will give you some indication of the awareness of the patient and the ability of the eyes to move into a correct position and use sight.

Questions 5.1 to 5.1.4
The questions on the position of the eyes.

Note the position of the eyes if they do not move. Apart from being in the middle, they may both look to one side, or else one eye may be in the middle and one looking to the outside, or else they may be separated and each looking towards the outside.

Abnormal eye position usually means that a part of the brain or one or more of the nerves working from the brainstem, responsible for the muscles which move the eye, has been damaged. This is usually the third cranial nerve, which is the main motor nerve to the muscles of the eye and which controls four of the six eye muscles.

Eyes usually do not remain fixed without some movement for more than a few days to a week, although a prolonged fixed eye can occur. It is important to decide when movement first occurs, and in what directions.

Questions 5.2.1 to 5.2.3
The questions on pupil size.

The size of our pupils determines how much light enters our eyes. If we enter a dark room, then our pupils enlarge or dilate, so we can take in more light and, therefore, see more. If we go into the sunlight, then our pupils constrict or grow smaller, to reduce the amount of light coming into the eye. If we are going into very strong sunlight, then we tend to wear a hat and sunglasses to reduce the input of light.

If the third cranial nerve to an eye is damaged from whatever cause, the pupil will tend to stay enlarged or dilated, even when a strong light is shone on to it and not infrequently the eyelid covering the enlarged pupil is also weak and may droop over the eye. The eye will often tend to look outwards. This may occur due to direct injury to the brain or the nerve or if the pressure inside the skull rises to an excessively high level.

Therefore, if, when you shine the light into the eye, there is no response, no constriction of the pupil, the patient is at STAGE 1 visually. You should mark it on the chart at the back of the Questionnaire.

STAGE 1   NO REACTION — PUPILS DO NOT CHANGE IN SIZE

STAGE 2   REFLEX STAGE

Questions 5.3.1 to 5.3.4.
Questions relating to the reaction of the pupil when you shine a 9-volt torch into the eyes.

If you can detect a change in the size of the pupil when you shine the light in, then the patient is at STAGE 2. You may sometimes need to use a magnifying glass and a strong light to check this out.

This means that light is entering the pupil, and while it may not be reaching the proper reception area of the brain (the visual cortex), it is at least going to one section where it can commence a reflex. This reflex constricts the pupil by using the third cranial nerve.

This does not mean that you can assume that vision is taking place.

This means that light is entering the eye. Mark the chart at Stage 2, if this occurs.

STAGE 3   WITHDRAWAL STAGE

Questions 5.4.1 and 5.4.2
When you touch the eyelid with your finger, does a blink occur?

The blink is a protective device for the eye by the eyelids which we use every day. If we are walking down the street and something hits our eyelids, we automatically close the lids, even before we have time to think about what has happened. It may be that this mechanism comes in very early, even in STAGE 2.

Questions 5.5.1 and 5.5.2
When you shine a strong torch into the eyes, does blinking occur?

This is also part of the protective mechanism with which we are all very familiar. If we walk out into strong sunlight or into a glare from strong lights, automatically we blink and may close our eyes. If this occurs with the patient, it may indicate that s/he is into STAGE 3. It also confirms that s/he is picking up the light from the environment.

Questions 5.6.1 and 5.6.2
When you move your finger towards the eye, does blinking occur?

If we see an object coming towards our eye and we anticipate that it will hit our eye, we will close our eyelids for protection. This is a reflex survival mechanism. If this consistently happens with the patient in coma, then you know that the patient has some vision, and is able to pick up the movement of your fingers towards the eyes. You must be sure that you do not touch the eye or eyelid when you do this test.

You will notice that the progression of stimuli you have used has been from

113

coarse to fine: it has been from touch to the eyelid, to light into the eye, to an object moving towards the eye. The ability of the eye to pick up an object moving towards it is a very much more sophisticated brain function than something touching the eyelid or a light shone in the eye.

If the answer to any of the questions in this section is yes, then you must mark Stage 3 on the visual section of Chart 1.

STAGE 4   THE LOCALIZING STAGE

Eye movement depends upon the functioning of six muscles attached to the sides of the eye that swing it from side to side and also in a vertical and rotatory direction. We need to be able to use this eye movement for two major purposes. We need to be able to move our eyes towards a stationary stimulus and fix on to it even if we are moving. We also need to be able to keep our eyes fixed on to a stimulus which moves while we are stationary, and pursue it during its movement.

Questions 5.7.1 and 5.7.2
Is there scanning?

The eye muscles which perform this eye movement can sometimes be damaged in head injury, but by far the most likely cause of the eye failing to be in the correct position, or failing to move correctly, is damage to the *nerves* serving these muscles. These nerves all come from the brainstem and are very likely to be involved if there is brainstem damage. They are the third, fourth and sixth cranial nerves.

Question 5.8
Do the eyes move together?

Scanning normally occurs with both eyes moving together. If the nerve to the muscle of an eye is damaged, then the muscle will not be able to move the eye properly. It is, therefore, unable to keep pace with the good eye and scan properly. You will feel it is like watching Marty Feldman. One eye will look one way and the other eye another.

We need to have our eyes moving together, so that the image from each eye goes to the correct place in our brain. If separate images go to our brain, then we either "see double", or we use one eye as a dominant eye, and neglect to use the other.

Question 5.9.1
Is there any movement of the eyes or head towards a visual stimulus?

Usually when something "catches our eye", we will turn our eyes towards it. In other words, we are "aware" of change in our environment and want to know what it is. If it is something which demands our attention, we will turn our eye and even swing our head towards it. We may even turn our whole body towards it, if necessary, depending upon the strength and importance of the stimulus to us. In other words we *localize* the stimulus. Our ancestors needed to do this to search for food and to defend themselves. The great Russian psychologist, Pavlov, called it the orienting reflex.

If the brain-injured patient can localize or orient, he is at the Localizing Stage or Stage 4. This means that he or she has an awareness of the environment which allows them to discriminate an object or person from that environment. In its early stages it is still a very primitive reaction.

Sometimes there may just appear to be a "drift" of the eyes towards the stimulus and then a drift off again. But this movement usually strengthens with time. Sometimes, the patient is unable to move the eyes towards a stimulus, or may only be able to move them in one direction. This may mean that there is evidence of awareness, but has damage to the part of the brain or nerves serving the muscles of the eye. It is most unlikely that the patient will move his head towards a visual stimulus in an early stage of coma.

Questions 5.10.1 to 5.10.6
Questions relating to whether you think the eyes look at a light, an object or a face.

The visual stimulus which is most easily identified by the brain appears to be white light: i.e, daylight or torchlight, etc. This is reasonable, as the most basic function for our eyes to perform is to detect the difference between night and day. Sometimes different colours have varying effects. It is worth trying the primary colours of red, yellow and blue. In our experience, after white light comes yellow, and then red, as effective stimuli.

Questions 5.11.1 to 5.11.6
Questions relating to whether you think the eyes follow a light, or an object, or a face?

Once the eyes have started to move towards a visual stimulus, you will generally find that this movement becomes stronger, more definite, more rapid, more easily provoked. You will get the impression that the eyes are now starting to "look at", take notice of, the stimulus.

How much notice is being taken of the stimulus by the patient is difficult to say, but this fixing of the eyes on to a stimulus is important. Because our brains seem to pick up light, this fixing usually occurs first on a white light and then on to an object, especially a bright one. Once again, it appears that the primary colours are best, with yellow and red the most effective. It is worth trying a variety of colours, however. When a patient can fix, and follow, on to a light or object, this usually means increasing awareness, which is what you are after, as well as increased visual function.

Once the eyes have scanned, identified that there is a light or object which is different from the rest of the environment, and fixed on to it, then the function of *localization* is established. Localizing on to a stationary stimulus is easier than localizing on to a moving stimulus. If the eyes of the patient will follow, or pursue, a light, or a face, or an object, eye function is becoming more effective. (Do not forget that if some of the nerves to the eye muscles have been damaged, then perhaps only one eye will be able to do these things, or else the eye or eyes may only be able to fix and pursue in the one direction.)

The ability to do any of the aspects of localization allows you to mark the visual chart at that level: that is STAGE 4.

STAGE 5   DISCRIMINATING STAGE

Questions 5.12.1 and 5.12.2
Do you think there is any eye contact between you and the patient?

What a delight it is, to have a patient look deep into your eyes, and you feel that contact has been established. As Michael Argyle sees it in his book *Social Encounters* (Penguin Books, 1973), when eye contact is present it is "signalling that the channel is open," i.e, the channel between your brain and the patient's brain.

He also writes in *The Psychology of Interpersonal Behaviour* (Penguin Books, 1967) that "Gaze is of central importance in human behaviour."

Up to now you may have had the impression that the patient was looking towards you, but the feeling was that they were looking "through" you, not into your eyes. When s/he looks into your eyes, you know that s/he is trying to connect his or her brain to yours.

What s/he has now done is localize you, discriminate your outline from the environment, move his or her eyes towards your face (we all look towards faces — even small infants are drawn to look at the face of their mother), identify the position of your eyes, and then look at them and into them.

First of all, this eye contact may be sporadic, and only for a fleeting period of time, at certain times of the day and perhaps only with special people. But then it becomes more established, more constant, more definite, more certain. Sometimes, in the early stages it will only appear when you demand it. I remember one patient who would not look at me until I pulled firmly on the hair on the right side of his head. Then he would look at me and communicate with me by grimace, indicating that I should stop. Once you have eye contact you have *discrimination*. Quite an effort for a person coming out of coma.

Questions 5.13.1 to 5.13.3
Does the patient appear to recognize photographs or pictures or people?

With time and effort, progress may continue until the person can finely discriminate pictures, words, etc.

If eye contact is occurring, mark Stage 5 on the visual part of Chart 1 at the end of the chapter.

---

6   AUDITORY FUNCTION

The response of the patient to sound is a measure of both general awareness, and ability to hear. Hearing seems to be one of the senses that "hangs in", even when other senses appear to be non-functioning. There are many recorded cases of people claiming to have heard all the conversation around their bed while they are regarded as being in coma. There is the story, probably apocryphal, of one comatose patient who, on recovery, considered that she had obtained enough information while in coma to enable her to live the rest of her life on the blackmail money extracted from the nurses talking around her bed!

The comatose patient seems to hear far more than we consider possible. That is why we are obsessive about being careful at the bedside, by telling the patient what you are doing, and making sure that no one utters any destructive comments.

The recovery of hearing goes through the same general hierarchical pattern as visual function. First, there is an awareness which is a very primitive reflex, which then passes on to the withdrawal stage, and then to the localizing or orienting stage, before moving into the stage of discrimination.

What you now need to find out is: Can the patient hear, and if so, how well, and can s/he understand or comprehend what is said? The questions in the section in hearing in the Questionnaire are designed to give you an idea of how aware the patient is, from the hearing point of view, and also to tell you what is the level of hearing ability and possibly understanding.

Question 6.1
Does the patient blink or move if you make a loud noise?

Once the first two weeks have passed after the accident, most families who are asked this question say they think the patient can hear. If you make a loud noise near the patient, does she or he jump or move their eyelids, or grimace, or does their breathing increase in speed, or do they breathe more deeply? If any of these things happen consistently, it is very likely that the patient can hear. This does not mean s/he understands. It is impossible to tell how much the patient hears, and what is understood, but all you are interested in with this question is, can the patient hear?

If, when you blow a horn or bang some wooden blocks together, there is no response in any way, then you must assume that the patient is either still deeply in coma (in unresponsive coma), or at that stage is deaf to noise. In my experience it is unusual to find a patient who does not give some response to noise, or to find a patient who is deaf from the brain injury.

Question 6.2
If you continue the noise, does the patient stop blinking or moving?

You must find out what happens to the patient when you make a loud noise and continue to do the same. In other words, you must blow the horn once, and then blow it again another four or five times. The patient may blink or give some other response as long as you continue to make the noise, or he may stop after five or six loud sounds. Some patients will stop blinking as you continue to make the noise. These patients we say have "habituated". Many patients will continue to blink or respond in other ways; these patients have not habituated.

Habituation really means that the noise has been picked up by the ear, the brain has heard the sound, in a primitive way has identified that it is no threat, and has "switched off", so that it does not respond to the sound any more.

If the patient habituates and you recommence the sound again after a short break, you will get the response again. Once a patient habituates, then this can be seen as a move from the Reflex Stage (Stage 2), up to the Withdrawal Stage (Stage 3).

Questions 6.3.1 and 6.3.2
Does the patient turn the eyes or head towards a noise?

The answer to this question will determine whether the patient has the ability to localize on to an auditory stimulus. In other words, can s/he find out where, or in what direction, the noise is. We all need to know if we are in danger, and our ears and hearing, being long-range detectors, must tell us where in space any unusual noise occurs which is a threat to our life.

If we hear something which is unusual, we may first of all turn our eyes towards it, and if we are concerned we may turn our head towards it, and if it really demands our attention, we will turn our whole body towards it. If the patient does this, s/he has the ability to localize and s/he has passed from the Withdrawal Stage (Stage 3) to the Localizing Stage (Stage 4).

Question 6.4
Does the patient appear to recognize a known voice?

Often relatives will note that the patient, even though still in coma, appears to react to different people in different ways. This is especially so if children are brought to the bedside. Many parents, who give little evidence of response, will react when their children are brought to the bedside and encouraged to talk to them, tell them what they are doing, what their school friends are doing, etc. Often the staff will also notice that one member of the nursing staff appears to get more response when they talk to the patient than any other. This is not to imply that the patient can understand what is being said to them, although this must always be considered to be so.

It is also important to note that a patient may be able to respond to a known voice, but still be unable to localize, if the nerves to the eye muscles are not yet working sufficiently, or if s/he is too weak to turn the head in the direction of the noise.

If the patient consistently recognizes a known voice, it is possible that the brain has gained more sophisticated function, and the patient is now able to discriminate, at least in a rough or coarse fashion. The patient may have passed into the Discriminating Stage (Stage 5).

Question 6.5
Does the patient appear to recognize the tone of the voice?

If a person is emotionally upset, and does not disguise this or hide it from the patient, the patient will often pick up this emotion of anxiety, or fear, or worry, and will respond with a look of anxiety on their face. It is very much as if the patient is tapping into the anxiety of the visitor and reflecting that. This is something which we all do when we meet people who are showing emotion, whether it is unhappiness, or happiness. We gauge their emotional tone. To do this, the patient must have some ability to be aware and discriminate.

Question 6.6
Will the patient relax if asked to do so?

This question ties in with the previous one. Often the patient who is uptight, or even in a spasm, will respond to someone who knows and loves him or her and will be comforted by their presence and their talking.

If the patient does relax when requested, once again it is not possible to know how much the patient understands, but you must regard him or her as being awake.

Question 6.7
Does the patient respond to words in an appropriate manner?

If the patient responds to words in an appropriate manner, there is no doubt that s/he has cortex or higher-brain function.

Often the patient is unable to give any indication that she or he can understand what is going on except by emotional expressions. If, when you are about to leave the patient's room, you say that you are going, and they look with anxiety or worry on their face, or start to breathe more deeply or rapidly, you must consider that they may understand what you are about to do.

Often relatives or friends will note that when the talk is about special things which are dear to the heart of the patient, s/he will respond. Those things which are closest to us all are our personal relationships, so the topics which are most likely to bring a response are those in which the family and close friends feature.

What children in the family are doing is especially important to parents, and the patient will often register on the face if either distressing or happy episodes are discussed. If this facial expression occurs repeatedly under a variety of different circumstances, you can consider that s/he understands words.

Question 6.8
Has the patient obeyed a command?

If the patient has obeyed a command, and this has been repeated and verified by more than one observer, the patient is out of coma. You will already be aware that there is a great deal of dispute about the endpoint of coma, but if you have asked the patient to move, and s/he has, then s/he must have higher-brain or cortex functioning.

There are three problems which will occur in confirming if a command has been obeyed or not:

Firstly, often the patient will move for relatives or friends, but will not move for the doctors or nurses.

Secondly, there is often a "time lag" between when the request is made, and when the patient carries out the command, and therefore you must make allowances for this.

Thirdly, actions can be misinterpreted. This applies especially to the request to squeeze a hand. There is what is known as a grasp reflex: it comes into action the moment you place your hand into the hand of the patient, who grasps automatically, and this is easily mistaken for a voluntary movement.

Another action which leads to confusion is to ask the patient to look at you. If they have reached the point where they can localize on to a visual stimulus, they may look at you at the same time by coincidence when you ask them.

One other area of confusion is where the patient has some movement of the arms or legs which is occurring spontaneously and without any apparent reason. If you ask the patient to move the leg and he or she does so randomly, at the same time, you may think that a command is being obeyed when it is not.

With perseverance, and without jumping to conclusions, it is possible to determine if the patient is obeying a command or not.

Do not forget what I said before about the variation in the patient's abilities from day to day and from time to time during the day. Never ever draw a conclusion on this matter from just one episode. Always look again and verify what you have seen.

---

7   TACTILE FUNCTION

What you need to find out from these questions is: "How much information is the patient getting into the brain from the touch environment?"

How aware is s/he of environmental inputs, can s/he localize where they are coming from, and can s/he discriminate what they are?

The patient who is brain-injured and does not respond to pain is deeply in coma. If the patient is only 1 on the Glasgow Coma Scale for the motor component, the prognosis is not good. Most patients who are on 1, and who survive, do not stay on 1. Usually, after a few days, the patient begins to show some response, which is called posturing: that is, when some stimulus is applied to the body, the whole of their body is committed to an action, often with the arms stretched out or sharply bent at the elbows and with the legs also stretched out. This is the Reflex Stage (Stage 2). (See Chapter 2: Measuring the Patient's Condition and What it Means.)

As the patient improves, this posturing is replaced by a withdrawal reaction, where the limb being touched is pulled away from the stimulus. This means that the patient is at the Withdrawal Stage (Stage 3).

As the condition of the patient improves further, s/he will be able to localize where the stimulus is on the body by either placing his or her hand or foot on to the stimulus. When s/he does this, s/he has passed into the Localizing Stage (Stage 4).

From there, as s/he regains more function, s/he will pass into the Discriminating Stage (Stage 5).

Question 7.1
Does the patient appear to feel pain?

Pain is the most demanding sense which our bodies can feel. If we have a severe toothache, it dominates our thoughts and actions. The same applies to a kidney stone or gout. Pain is a signal to our bodies that there is danger directly encroaching on our "intimate space". That demands our attention. The closer the threat, the more the danger.

If the patient does not respond to pain, s/he is very deeply in coma: that is, No Response (Stage 1).

Question 7.2.1 and 7.2.2
Does the patient appear to feel heat or cold?
Does the patient relax in the bath?

Temperature changes do not demand as quick a response from us as pain, unless they are severe enough to cause pain. Therefore, to be able to pick up temperature changes of heat or cold indicates a more responsive patient than the one who can only pick up pain.

The response to cold can be easily tested by putting some ice on to a limb, or on to the chest, or abdomen, and watching the result.

It is possible, however, to get the withdrawal reflex where a limb is moved away from the stimulus, and this means that the patient is in the Withdrawal Stage.

Sometimes, when the ice is placed on the abdomen, the patient will reach out and attempt to knock it off, even while s/he appears to be comatose. This indicates that the patient is in the Localizing Stage.

Testing the response to heat can present a problem. Hospitals are quite rightly very wary of applying heat to a patient, since too many patients have been accidentally burnt, which can constitute negligence. I do not think it is wise to place anything hot on the patient.

One way of finding out if the patient responds to heat is to ask if the patient relaxes in a warm bath. If this does occur, you at least know the patient is responding to heat. It is also worth asking if the patient jumps if splashed with cold water, to confirm any work you have done with an ice-pack.

Question 7.3
Does the patient become more aware when touched?

While pain is the most demanding of the stimuli when applied to our body, followed by heat or cold, touch can also bring about a response in a patient. This usually only occurs after there are good responses to pain and cold. Touch, especially light touch from someone whom we know, is more soothing than demanding. Often you will find that the patient will become more relaxed if touched, or massaged, by a familiar person. If this occurs, then you know that the patient is capable of picking up touch sensation.

121

Question 7.4
Does the patient appear to register discomfort?

We all seek a comfortable position. If we can't find one, we wriggle until we can, or until we can move our body to another more comfortable place. All animals do this. The cat finds the most comfortable chair in the house, and the dog seeks out the sun near the kennel.

The patient who is brain-injured, but who is capable of registering discomfort, reacts similarly. S/He will wriggle in an effort to reduce the discomfort. This means that somewhere inside the brain there is the knowledge that the body needs a new position. It is worth noting whether the patient moves from his or her back to the side or vice versa, or pulls the legs up or stretches them out.

Some patients wriggle so much they are tied in a chair, but their body language is saying "let me out".

You must be careful in interpreting the meaning of any movement. If the patient is deeply in coma, he or she may reflexly move into a fixed position: arms and legs often either bent up or stretched out. If he or she constantly moves into these positions, do not take this as evidence of registering discomfort or of awareness.

Question 7.5
Does the patient react in any way when his body or limbs are moved?

Patients who are deeply comatose will not respond when body or limbs are moved. As s/he becomes more awake, however, s/he may start to open the eyes, grimace or breathe heavily or rapidly when they are moved. There are actually many channels of sensation being stimulated by that movement, some of them very old. There are the sensations which are involved with balance and position, the sensations which are involved with joint and muscle movement, and the sensations of touch. Because the head is also moved at the same time, there may also be visual sensations as the eyes are moved with the head. Body and limb movement is, therefore, very important. While at first the patient may react with the whole body (that is, s/he will "posture" when s/he is first moved), this reaction tends to reduce slowly with time.

The explanations relating to *Questions 7.6.1 to 7.10.1* are dealt with in the motor response section on the Glasgow Coma Scale in Chapter 2. It is worth while checking on this section again.

Questions 7.11.1 to 7.11.6
Can the patient tell you about an object by touching?

If the patient can tell whether an object is large or small, hot or cold, soft or hard by touch, s/he is out of coma and has the ability to use touch to discriminate different objects.

CHAPTER 12

ASSESSING THE RETURN OF MOTOR OUTPUT

We will deal here with Questions 8 to 20 relating to the return of motor function.

After brain injury, it is difficult to predict the motor functions which will be totally or partially lost.

Just as sensations return in an ordered manner, so do the muscle functions. You will have noted already that there is a sequence which is followed as sensations return. There is also a sequence as motor function returns.

The Requirements for Motor Function

All muscle function has certain things in common. These functions are easily remembered if you think of a gun emplacement. Both muscles and guns work for a specific purpose, that is, to hit the target. With both muscles and guns, failure to hit the target is failure of function.

A gun needs:

1. *Stability*. A stable base from which to fire. If the gun is unstable or wobbly, then all aspects of the function of firing are jeopardized, and failure to hit the target will occur.

2. *Mobility*. Mobility is needed so that the position and direction of fire can be altered. Failure to change direction limits the gun to a fixed field of fire, which places gross limitations on the position of the targets which can be hit. This is reminiscent of the guns operating in World War II in Singapore, which pointed fixedly out to sea and could not be swung into position to deal with the attacking forces from the rear.

3. *Distance and Power*. Power to be able to fire the correct distance is essential if a target is to be hit. Charges which fall short of the target are non-functional. Charges which have expended their energy when they hit the target are of no value.

4. *Feedback*. Feedback is necessary from an observer, so that direction, distance or power can be modified and the target hit.

Underlying the whole of this process of firing the gun is the intention and motivation to hit the target. In addition, there must be the coordination of sequences, so that the complex actions required can be arranged in correct sequence.

Muscle function is the same as firing a gun. It needs;

1. A stable base from which to work.

2. Mobility to change direction.
3. Correct distance in the movement, and correct strength to gain the desired effect.
4. Feedback to ensure that it has performed the action correctly.

Failure of any of these factors in regard to muscle will produce failure of the desired movement, just as failure of any of the factors with a gun and its emplacement will mean that the target will not be hit.

The Sequence of Recovery of Motor Function

There appear to be five major stages which the brain-injured person goes through in an effort to regain muscle function. These stages are:

STAGE 1   NO REACTION
STAGE 2   REFLEX MOVEMENT
STAGE 3   SPONTANEOUS MOVEMENT
STAGE 4   CONTROLLED MOVEMENT
STAGE 5   FINE CONTROLLED MOVEMENT

These will be dealt with in this chapter and linked with the questionnaire.

---

8   *STAGE 1   NO MOVEMENT — POSITION*

Question 8.1.1
Does the patient move any part of the body?

The patient who is deeply in coma may have no movement capability of his or her own, and will tend to fix into a specific type of posture. This fixed posture is usually of two types.

Questions 8.2.1 to 8.2.4
If the patient does not move, what is her/his position?

The Arms

The Flexed Position. If the arms are bent at the elbows, then the position is known as flexed. Often when the arms are flexed, the elbows tend to be close together on the chest and the wrist and fingers bent. This position has been already discussed in Chapter 2. It indicates that the patient has a generalized reaction to a stimulus and is functioning at a primitive brain level. It is classed as 3 on the motor part of the Glasgow Coma Scale.

The Extended Position. The arms are stretched out, usually with the palms showing backwards or else away from the body and the fingers outstretched. This has also been dealt with in Chapter 2, and indicates that there is a generalized response showing that primitive brain function is being used. It is even more primitive than the flexed position. It is classed as 2 on the motor part of the Glasgow Coma Scale.

The Legs

The Flexed Position. The position of the legs may also vary. Where the legs are bent at the hips and knees, the position is known as flexed.

The Extended Position. The hips and knees may be stretched out with the feet and toes pointing down. This is called extended.

In general, it is considered that the extended position, especially of the arms, indicates worse damage than the flexed position.

It is unusual for a patient to remain in these abnormal positions without any movement for weeks or months. The longer a patient does remain in these positions without movement, the worse must be considered the prognosis.

Most patients who initially have no movement, gain reflex movements in the weeks or months following the brain injury.

---

9   STAGE 2   REFLEX MOVEMENT

Sometimes the first movements are what are termed *spasms*. These are a jerky movement the patient makes, usually when disturbed. The spasm movement is a total body one, with the arms and legs bending into flexion or stretching into extension, all at the one time. Spasms are common. No one likes to see them, and everyone is relieved when they pass, which they usually do with time.

It is frequently difficult to decide on the factors which produce a spasm. Stimuli in the environment can be the initiating cause. The predisposing cause, or the reason why the brain is set up to produce the spasm is still a cause of conjecture. In other words, how much of the spasm is due to the problems with the internal homeostasis and how much is due to the external environment is unknown. For the purposes of this book, spasms are regarded as reflex movements which arise from a brain which is damaged and are often brought about through the stimuli in the environment.

Question 9.1
Are there any reflex movements?

In Chapter 2, "Measuring the Patient's Condition and What it Means", the reflex movements are dealt with as measured by the Glasgow Coma Scale, in the motor response section. All movements scaled as 2 and 3 are classed as total body reflex movements, while those classed as 4 are local reflex movements or withdrawal.

To put it another way, the reflex movements can be seen when a stimulus is applied to the head, limbs or body. They can vary from spasms of the entire body, which we have called total body movement, to local withdrawal of the part of the body or limb being stimulated.

It is important, therefore, for you to understand that there is a tremendously wide range of reflex movements which have a great variation also in significance, the total body movements being the most primitive and the most worrying.

Question 9.1.1
Is the reflex movement a total body movement? (i.e, marked 2 or 3 on the Glasgow Coma Scale)

In some patients the total body movement is so strong that the back will arch, and the person will actually lift the back off the bed like a bridge, a condition known as opisthotonus.

In others, the type of total body movement will be either the extension or flexion type movement described in Chapter 2.

Some total body movements are a composite of these two states.

Question 9.1.2
How strong are the total body reflex movements?

The spasms may be classified as strong, moderate or weak. Strong spasms can be easily observed, for the body movement will be very definite.

Weak spasms are sometimes even difficult to detect. If there is total body commitment, it must still be regarded as a spasm. Of course, anything between strong and weak can be classified as moderate.

Question 9.1.3
How long do the total body movements last?

Obviously strong spasms are worrying, especially if they continue for a long period of time. They vary tremendously from being only momentary and lasting for a few seconds to where they last for minutes.

I can recall one boy, Stephen, who had intense spasms for almost two months. These slowly passed off. He had tremendous family support. His family was told to place him in a nursing home, but he is now at home and has just started at a special education school. Mentally, he is very bright. Physically, he has major deficiencies of speech, hand function and mobility, but in all these he is slowly improving.

Questions 9.1.4 and 9.1.5
How frequent are the total body movements?
What brings them on?

If strong spasms occur frequently, sometimes several in an hour, they are of more significance than if they only occur once per day.

They can be brought on by the stimuli of noise, touch, light, movement, pain, etc,. If they are brought on by slight stimuli, this is more worrying than when a great deal of stimulation is required to produce them.

Questions 9.1.6 and 9.1.7
Can you stop the spasms?

This is often difficult to answer at first. You may talk to the patient or stroke the patient, and she/he will stop the spasm, but it is often difficult to be sure that this was not coincidence. If, however, you feel that repeatedly you or someone else can stop the spasms by talking or touching the patient, this may be seen of great benefit and your answer to this question should be yes.

If you can stop the spasms, this indicates that the patient is receptive to either your touch or your voice or a combination of both and has sensory input. It also indicates that in some manner he/she is capable of reducing or controlling the spasms.

Question 9.2
Is the reflex a local withdrawal?

If placing ice or causing pain on one limb results in movement or withdrawal only of that limb and the other limbs remain still, the reflex is a local one. The significance of this is dealt with in Chapter 2 in the motor section of the Glasgow Coma Scale. A strong movement is welcome — the stronger the better.

---

10   STAGE 3   SPONTANEOUS MOVEMENTS

Spontaneous movements are great. The patient may move his head or an arm or leg without you touching him. It is impossible to be sure of exactly what is going on, but in my experience spontaneous movements are indications that recovery is occurring. It is an exciting thing when a patient, having had spasms, or only reflex movements, makes a spontaneous movement.

Often the movement first comes when the patient is put in water, in the bath or in a spa. When it comes it is like gold.

Questions 10.1.1 and 10.1.2
Are there any spontaneous movements of the head?

I have already stressed the importance of the head. It is the only part of the body which contains the sense organs of the eyes, ears, taste and smell — and also has some elements of touch.

It has the long-range receptors for vision and hearing and the receptor of smell. We need to be able to move our head to allow us to direct our senses, or localize on to stimuli in the environment.

The movements of the head which you need to know about are in two major directions. The first is a rotation or turning of the head to either side. The second is the lifting movement of the head upwards. Usually the patient's head drops forward on to the chest, and there is difficulty in lifting it up. Since the head weighs about 3 kilograms in an adult, this is not surprising.

It is the rotary movement which usually comes in first; the head-lifting movement may take months to come. This rotation of the head is usually first seen when the patient is lying down with the back of the head supported on a pillow. The movement is often very slight at first, but develops with time and use.

Remember, it is usually difficult for the patient to move her or his head if it is set heavily into pillows, or there is a sandbag on each side of the head to stop movement.

It is also a common finding that the patient can rotate the head if sitting up in a chair with the back of the head supported.

Sometimes, the head appears to be held firmly, facing in one direction. It is as if the muscles of the neck have contracted or tightened on one side, and have released on the other. The head, therefore, tends to lie in one position, and no movement in the other direction occurs. Given time and work, this fixed state of affairs often passes, and weak movement begins to rotate the head.

It is frequently difficult to be sure what causes the head to move. In fact, it is very likely that, even though you do not know, the patient is attempting to localize or discriminate something in the environment. Often the patient will turn the head towards a source of light, like the window or towards the electric light in the room, or will turn the head to where the sound is most intense, such as a door opening on to a corridor where there is activity, such as people moving along and making a noise.

It is sometimes difficult to tell if the movement is controlled and, therefore, Stage 4 or still only spontaneous and in Stage 3. This problem is not of any significance and commonly passes with time and further observation.

Question 10.2
Are there any spontaneous movements of the body? Does the patient wriggle and change his/her position?

Everyone becomes uncomfortable just lying in bed and not changing position. When we sleep, we all change our position from lying on our side or our back or our front. Even if we are lying in the sun on the beach, we only maintain the one position for a relatively short time, and then move, either wriggling into the sand or raising ourselves on an elbow, or shifting from side to side.

If the patient has an awareness of body touch, and is aware of the position of muscles and joints, s/he also must feel uncomfortable staying in the same place without movement and change of position.

It is, therefore, important to note if the patient wriggles or gives some other indication that she or he can change position. If they can, it implies that they have some body power which, while it may be weak and limited, is better than no power at all.

In the very early stages the only way this body movement might be seen is to lie the patient on their side, at a point of balance, and see if they can roll either on to the back or the front.

You must always be aware that nursing staff turn these patients frequently and, therefore, a change of position must be seen happening, not after it has been completed.

Questions 10.3 and 10.4
Are there any spontaneous movements of the right or left arms?

In my experience limbs usually move before the head, unless the patient has a special type of injury, or the limb is confined by splints or plasters. The easiest way for you to chart limb movement is to use the concept of the personal zones which was given in Chapter 6. You will recall that the intimate zone was the one which involved the space around the body surface itself. What you want to know is: what is the range of movement of each arm on to that body surface. The places to be charted are the head, face, chest, abdomen, groin and leg.

It is most likely that the arm is positioned on the abdomen (stomach). It may move spontaneously upwards onto the chest or down towards the groin. Downward movement is often indicated, if you find that the catheter into the bladder or the urodome is pulled by the patient. If removal of the catheter by the patient has occurred, the range of spontaneous movement must have increased.

The catheter does represent an irritating stimulus for the patient, and this will draw their attention. Sometimes catheters just fall out, so you need to have more than one episode where the catheter or urodome is out of position, or you need to see the hand of the patient extended to the catheter before you can conclude that they have increased the range of movement.

The likely upward movement is the attempted removal of the nasogastric tube. It is not unusual for the patient to attempt to remove this which indicates the ability to move the arm on to the face. Movement of the arm into a higher position on to the head can also occur. I recall one young male, who, according to his mother, had been quite vain before the accident and was for ever brushing his hair. His hand frequently went up on to his head.

Movement out of the intimate zone is seen if the arm of the patient stretches out to the side or into a forward position. S/he may also pick up one hand with the other. These movements usually only occur when the patient is recovering a significant amount of function.

Often you will find that the patient can move only one arm and the other is not capable of spontaneous movement. While it is nice to have both arms moving, it is at least a good sign that one can move.

Even the slow arm, or the arm which does not move, can gradually commence movement, and it is interesting to watch the pattern of recovery of the slow arm, which tends to be in a similar manner to the arm which has led recovery.

Question 10.5
Are there any spontaneous movements of the right or left leg?

Movement in the legs often appears before movement in the arms. The legs are not great guardians of the intimate zone, but total body movement away from threat is dependent upon our legs and is of immense importance to all people. Without leg function we are very dependent upon others. Normally, the leg is not as mobile as the arm. The joints of the leg at the hip and knee and ankle provide for stability, not mobility. The major movements of the legs are the back-and-forth or up-and-down movements of walking. It is this up-and-down movement you look for, to see spontaneous movements in the lower limbs. Often you see movements of the toes before you see any major joints, such as the hip or knee, being moved.

Question 10.6
Is there any tremor?

All of the spontaneous movements may appear to us to be aimless. They are often unco-ordinated and may appear to be quite jerky. It is worth while noting if the movement has a definite shake or tremor. Sometimes, because the patient is weak, the movement may appear shaky, but usually with time the shakiness goes. If, however, the tremor is constant, you should take note of it. It may be present only when the patient moves the limb, or it may be present when the patient has the limb at rest. You may also see a tremor in the eyes of the patient. Since tremor is a very complicated subject you should ask your doctor about its significance.

---

11 STAGE 4 CONTROLLED MOVEMENT

What a relief it is when the patient will voluntarily move their head or body or a limb when you ask them to do so. This ability to obey a command, or a request, repeatedly is taken as an indication that the coma has ceased and the patient is awake. If you go back to Chapter 8, you will see that coming out of coma, the endpoint of coma, is taken as the ability to obey a command or request.

Do not forget the difficulty which the medical staff have in deciding the endpoint of coma, especially if they are in a hurry, or rush their examination, or ask the patient to do things which s/he cannot do. Remember, there is no point in asking the patient to demonstrate that s/he is out of coma by asking them to move their right hand if, all s/he can do is move their left leg. So you must be careful. You must ask the patient to perform the function which they can accomplish.

If the patient has voluntary movement, what you are about to do is to chart out the extent of function and the extent of disability.

The questions in Stage 4 are identical to those with assessing spontaneous movement. The only difference is that the patient is being checked to see if he or she can voluntarily control their movement.

In each one of these movements the factors which I spoke about in regard to the gun emplacement apply. Because of their importance I will repeat and slightly enlarge what I stated at the beginning of the chapter. All movement has a target. For that target to be reached, the factors involved are:

1. A stable base.
2. A freedom to move the limb in the correct direction.
3. Ability to move the limb the correct distance.
4. The right amount of force.
5. Co-ordination.
6. The least expenditure of energy.
7. The correct speed.
8. A feedback mechanism to correct for any changes in the objective or the wishes of the person.

The patient you are charting has been extremely ill. She or he will not regain all

130

abilities suddenly. Their movements will be coarse, and often uncontrolled to a great degree.

When you first look and assess, you just want to know what the patient can do. The niceties of how they do it can be observed over time, as they regain more of these abilities, and powers of fine tuning come in.

Questions 11.1.1 and 11.1.2
Will s/he obey a request to move the head?

If the patient obeys a request to move their head, you need to know in what direction. Can they rotate it both ways? Can they lift the head up, if it is sagging on their chest? If they can do these things, it is very likely that they can also keep their head balanced in the upright position without it flopping to one side or the other or falling forward.

Question 11.2.1
Does the patient wriggle or change position if asked to do so?

Sometimes patients will obey a request to wriggle or move position more easily than to move a limb. This is especially so if they have fractures of their bones or if they have inhibition plasters on the limbs.

Questions 11.3.1 to 11.4.10.
Will the patient obey a request to move his/her right or left arm?

Still use the idea of body space zones to identify what are the active ranges of movements of the arms of the patient. All the time you are really asking the patient how well are his/her protective abilities. You know, of course, that the movements will be very weak to commence with, but time and usage will strengthen them.

The big thing about arms is that they have hands on the end of them. Without good arm movement, hand usage is extremely limited. Without hand movement the arm is almost non-functional. You need to know what the patient can do with his or her arms, so you can see what the possibility is for hand function. Often you will find that the position in the bed or a chair will affect the range of movement, so see if there is a change of function when you place the patient in different positions.

Obviously, if you can chart the patient while they are making use of gravity, movement may be seen as both stronger and have a greater range. Conversely if they are working against gravity, movement becomes more difficult. So vary the position and ask them to do the same movements and note down the result.

Questions 11.5.1 to 11.5.4.
Will the patient obey a request to move his/her right or left leg?

You need the same sort of knowledge about the movement of the patient's legs and toes. Can he or she move them voluntarily, and under what conditions and what circumstances. It may be easier for him or her to move their legs when sitting on the edge of the bed. Sometimes if you start swinging the legs the patient may be able to keep it up. Sometimes the movement may occur when lying in bed. Note all these things down.

12 FINE CONTROLLED MOVEMENT

Gradually with use, hopefully the power and the direction and the mobility of motor function will return. It may never reach the same excellence which was present before the accident but change and improvement can occur for years after the accident. Do not give up attempting to get a better result until you feel that you have done the utmost.

13 HAND FUNCTION

Hand function is so important that I have a separate section for it. Recovery of hand function also goes through the previously described stages of:

STAGE 1	NO REACTION
STAGE 2	REFLEX MOVEMENT
STAGE 3	SPONTANEOUS MOVEMENT
STAGE 4	CONTROLLED MOVEMENT
STAGE 5	FINE CONTROLLED MOVEMENT

STAGE 1   NO MOVEMENT

Questions 13.1.1 and 13.1.2
Is there any movement of the hands?

Often the patient who is severely brain-injured has no grasp reflex. This primitive reflex is most easily seen in babies and infants. When you place a finger in the hand of a baby, the baby tends to close their hand on your finger, and hang on so tightly that you may have difficulty pulling your finger away. This is the grasp reflex.

With the patient who has no grasp reflex, when you place your finger or hand in theirs you will feel that there is no tension in the fingers. If you lift your hand up, his hand will fall away immediately. It is not uncommon for patients to be without this reflex. It usually returns after a few weeks.

STAGE 2   REFLEX MOVEMENT

Questions 13.2.1 and 13.2.2
Does the hand hold yours, when you place your hand in his/her palm?

The very weakest grasp reflex occurs when you place your fingers into the hand of the patient, whose hand is lying on the bed. As you slowly lift your hand up, you notice that their hand does not fall away immediately, but there appears to be some grasp or tension. This may, initially, be so weak that it is hard to be sure of it. And, of course, it can vary immensely from day to day and at different times of the day. It can also be affected by heavy drug therapy.

It is also possible, and indeed frequent, to have a marked variation between the right and left hand, depending upon the site and extent of the brain injury. This does not depend on whether the patient is right-handed or left-handed.

STAGE 3 SPONTANEOUS MOVEMENT

Questions 13.3.1 to 13.3.4
Does the index finger point?
Do the fingers open?

This is really asking, does the patient have a release mechanism for the hand? If you are a monkey up a tree, it is all very well to be able to grasp, but if you cannot let go, you are history.

We all need the ability to let go, just as much as we need the ability to grasp. Often this release mechanism takes a long time to come. An indication that it is developing is when the hand of the patient slowly starts to lose that very tight clenched-fist look, and the fingers open up slightly.

One of the indicators that this is developing more fully may be what one of my nurses, Maureen, termed the E.T. sign, from the movie *E.T. — The Extra-Terrestrial*. This sign occurs when a finger, usually the second finger, starts to straighten out and point. Sometimes the third finger will then join the second finger and point.

STAGE 4 CONTROLLED MOVEMENT

Question 13.4.1 to 13.4.3
Can the patient take something in their palm and hold it? Can they also release their grasp voluntarily?

If the patient can, on request, take something in their hand and hold it and release it, they have voluntary movement. Often this movement is very primitive initially, and the grip is not by finger and thumb, but between the palm and the other fingers. Obviously also, it may be very weak and unco-ordinated, but if it is present, it is extremely important in demonstrating the recovery process.

Questions 13.5.1 and 13.5.2
Can the patient take something between the finger and thumb?

To be able to take an object between the finger and thumb is to have higher brain function and indicates an ability to discriminate, and possibly develop, fine controlled movement, which is one of the important abilities of the human.

We really come back to the Glasgow Coma Scale again here *(Questions 14.1 to 14.4)*. Refer back to the section in Chapter 2.

The use of words in any form is an indication of higher brain function. The patient in coma may not make any sound, but when the recovery process moves under way, sound often occurs.

Obviously, if the patient has a tracheostomy, there is little or no air going past the vocal cords, and the making of a sound becomes impossible. If the patient is out of coma, they may commence to mouth words, that is, they may actually move their lips in an attempt to speak, even though no sound comes.

Once the tracheostomy tube is out, and the wound in the neck is closed, at least the air is able to flow past the cords and sounds may be made. At first, these may be only a groan, or a cry, but often speech does follow, even though it may take months or even years to come.

At first the speech consists of single words. The words frequently used are swear words, and they often come at times of great emotion. Over time the patient may start to join words together and formulate sentences.

Once words are being used, you know the patient is out of coma.

---

15   SWALLOWING

Question 15.1
Is there much saliva?

Patients with severe brain injury often have a great deal of saliva dribbling from their mouths which may require constant sucking out. This saliva may be due to excessive production, or to lack of ability to swallow, or to both. This dribbling tends to reduce as the patient regains swallowing.

Question 15.2
Can the patient swallow?

Swallowing is controlled by nerves at the lower part of the brainstem. As you are aware, damage to the brainstem may be one of the prime causes of coma and swallowing may be also affected.

Often the first sign of the return of swallowing is when there appears to be a reduction in the amount of saliva dribbling from the mouth of the patient. Swallowing is of extreme importance, for if normal feeding is to be eventually regained, it is dependent upon this function.

Question 15.3
Does she or he cough?

Since coughing safeguards our air passages from any foreign substances, the cough reflex is of great importance. You will find that no one will attempt to feed the patient until a cough reflex is re-established, and rightly so.

CONCLUSION

There is still much to be learnt about the patient coming out of coma. What I have attempted to do is formulate an approach. Like all early exploratory work there is always room for change. However, with the information obtained from the questionnaire, and the explanatory chapters, it is possible to determine into which basic category of coma the patient should be placed, and at what level of therapy the patient should be commenced and maintained.

Every week the questionnaire should be dated and redone, using different coloured ink, up to a maximum of four colours. Several photostats of the original should be kept and used over the months, if necessary.

All documentation should be kept in a book or folder, so you have a record of the progress of the patient. The same people, if possible, who did the initial assessments should be involved in those which follow, although this may be difficult at times.

With the changing condition of the patient, the programme provided will also need to be modified and made more sophisticated. At some stage also, hopefully, when the patient goes to rehabilitation, this document will be of great importance to the medical, nursing and paramedical staff.

The other method of recording which is valuable and should be used to supplement the written record is the use of video. Video records should all be classified with date, time, condition of the patient and name of the operator, so they can be used in a combined way with the other information.

ALL RECORDS SHOULD BE KEPT IN A SAFE PLACE.

SECTION D

HOW THE BRAIN FUNCTIONS

CHAPTER 13

SOME RULES OF BRAIN FUNCTION

This is not meant to give you a detailed account of how the brain works. Present knowledge of brain function does not allow this to be done adequately.

What is known, however, is that the brain is a very commonsense organ. The actions which we take, and which we see people do every day in our environment, are a reflection of our thinking, and their thinking, and therefore tell us a great deal about how our brains work.

It is important for you to to understand what is happening as the patient tries to regain brain function. It is important for you to know some of the ways in which the normal brain works.

The brain needs to get *information* IN and the brain needs to get *information* OUT. This IN — OUT mechanism is essential, if the brain is to work. Reduce or delete either section of the IN — OUT loop, and the brain cannot function to an optimum. It is important for you to go back to Chapter 4 and look once again at the cybernetic loop.

Many would liken this function on information to a computer. Computers do not, however, have a hot brain, and the comparison is limited because of the important and often overriding role that our emotions play through the hot brain.

There are rules which the brain follows at all times. I will use an everyday example of an interchange between people to demonstrate some of these rules.

A. The Stimulus-Response Mechanism

The brain works on what is called a *stimulus-response* mechanism. By that, I mean the brain needs to be able to detect in the environment any change (the stimulus) which occurs. It then needs to respond to the change (the response).

For this stimulus-response mechanism to work properly, the first thing needed is some awareness of the environment. We need to be at least partially conscious, awake and attentive.

The great Russian neuropsychologist, Aleksandr Luria, formerly Professor of Psychology at Moscow University and a member of the Academy of Pedagogical Sciences, wrote in *The Working Brain* (Penguin, 1973):

"For human processes to follow their correct course, the waking state is essential. It is only under optimal waking conditions that;
Man can receive and analyse information,
Man can call to mind the necessary selective system of connections,
He can programme his activities,

He can check the course of his mental processes,
He can correct his mistakes,
He can keep his activity to the proper course."
Let me illustrate what the stimuli and the responses are in a given situation.

In the City of Wells, in the United Kingdom, I was asleep in a hotel. The time was about two o'clock in the morning. There was a gentle knocking sound on one of the hotel doors, which lasted for about five seconds and stopped. The knocking was very gentle. It was enough to wake me up, but I was unknown in the hotel and the town and I therefore felt that it had no relevance to me. I rolled over and started to go back to sleep.

The knocking started again. It was now slightly louder. It went for longer. Only then did I start to wonder what was happening. The knocking changed to a banging. The person at the door had started to thump with his fist. I got out of bed and went to the window, for the thumping was now becoming very loud and aggressive. I looked out the window and saw a man standing at the door.

Just then he walked away from the door, lifted his head up towards the windows and called out in a loud angry voice. "Can't somebody in this hotel hear me. I have left my wallet with my passport, inside this hotel." At that time the hotel proprietor opened the door and let him in. Within a short period, the wallet retrieved, the man came out and left the hotel. I went back to sleep.

Let us look at what can be learnt from this simple set of actions (stimuli) and reactions (response).

The first thing that the man at the door had to do was wake us up and gain our attention: he had to provide a stimulus which changed the environment. He did this in three ways.

Firstly, he used his fingers and knocked at the door, providing an auditory stimulus (hearing) in the environment. This brought no response which he could detect.

Secondly, because he had given a stimulus but had no response from that stimulus, he increased the strength of the auditory stimulus by banging on the door with his fist, louder, more frequently and longer: he increased the intensity and the frequency and the duration of his stimulus. Even with this increase in his stimulus he still had not gained a response.

Thirdly, he walked away from the door, and changed the stimulus to one which was more demanding. He called out loudly. Then he gave additional stimuli by identifying himself and saying what his difficulty was.

A response then occurred. The proprietor, who was sleeping in the rear section of the hotel, woke up, realized that someone wanted him at his front door, walked to the door, let the man in, gave him his wallet, and the caller was then on his way to his next encounter with his environment.

Once a satisfactory response had occurred, the cycle of the stimulus-response loop had been completed and the man moved off into a new environment.

This stimulus-response loop is basic to the way our brains work.

We can assume that, if the proprietor had not appeared when the man at the door had called out, the caller would have changed his stimulus again and might have increased its intensity by banging on the door harder, calling out louder, and even kicking on the door. If this had failed, and he still wished to obtain his wallet, he might have gone to a phone booth and rung up the hotel or even gone to the police for help. *All to get a response.*

So we learn that, once our brain gives a stimulus to the environment, it demands a response. If we don't obtain the response which we want, we may become frustrated and angry.

The next thing we learn is that we don't give a response without a stimulus. It is highly unlikely that the proprietor would have woken up, got out of bed and walked to the door without a stimulus being given to him. It is highly unlikely that I would have woken out of my sleep and walked to the window and looked at the entrance door of the hotel without the stimulus from the caller. If that man had realized that he had left his wallet in the hotel, but decided that he would get it when the hotel opened in the morning, none of the above scene would have occurred.

So it is important to consider the following rules, which apply equally to the brain-injured and the non-brain-injured person. You do not need to learn them. You are familiar with them from general living. Just use them in your dealing with the brain-injured person.

RULE 1

WITHOUT A STIMULUS THERE WILL BE NO RESPONSE. The whole of this scene would not have occurred, if there had been no knock at the door in the first place.

RULE 2

AN *EFFECTIVE* STIMULUS IS NEEDED IF AN ADEQUATE RESPONSE IS TO BE PRODUCED. The stimulus will need to be strong enough to be effective. Tapping at the door was an ineffective stimulus.

RULE 3

THE STIMULUS MAY NEED TO BE *INTENSIFIED* IF THERE IS NO ADEQUATE RESPONSE. The caller intensified his stimulus to loud knocking at the door of the hotel.

RULE 4

THE STIMULUS MAY NEED TO BE *CHANGED* IF THERE IS NO ADEQUATE RESPONSE. The type of stimulus may need to be altered if there is not an adequate response. When knocking produced no response, the caller changed the stimulus to a vocal one by shouting.

RULE 5

FOR A PERSON TO RESPOND THERE MUST BE SOME *AWARENESS*. If the proprietor had continued to sleep, the stimulus-response cycle could not have occurred. The first thing needed to obtain an effective response was for the proprietor to awaken.

RULE 6

WE RESPOND TO THOSE THINGS WHICH *MATTER* TO US. I was closer to the door than the proprietor, but the matter was not one of my concern. I took no effective action.

RULE 7

IF WE GET NO RESPONSE, WE BECOME FRUSTRATED. THIS LEADS TO ANGER. The man at the door started off with his cold brain working. When he obtained no response, he became angry and his hot brain started to work. He became frustrated and angry.

B. The processing of information

The stimulus-response mechanism is basic to all brain function. The example given above used a very simple set of circumstances. Little of our living is involved in simple stimulus-response mechanism. Most living is a great deal more complicated.

Let me illustrate again. Most people are familiar with the problems of driving on a new freeway from which they have to exit at a specific point. Most freeway exits are well marked, but even so it is still possible to miss the turn-off. This situation occurred to me in the U.K. recently on the M1. Once again we must consider the key word: INFORMATION. I wanted to know where to leave the freeway to reach my destination. I had therefore to look for the critical signs which would allow my intention to be fulfilled.

I am used to driving on the left side of the road. No doubt things would have been worse if I normally drove on the right side of the road. I was not used to the speed of the traffic on the freeway and had difficulty controlling my speed to the pace at which I normally drive, with so many cars moving rapidly behind me and then passing me.

I was whizzing by the signs notifying the exits. My wife was having great difficulty reading them. I remonstrated with her about her inability to read the signs and give me the right directions. She told me very clearly that I was going too fast for her to see the signs and allow me time to pull off. She told me to slow down. I slowed down, approached the exit signs and gave her the opportunity of obtaining the information from them.

We noticed several things which would also be known to you. The bigger signs were easier to read than the smaller ones, the well-lit signs were easier to read than the poorly lit ones, the brightly coloured signs were easier to read than the dull ones, the signs which occurred more frequently made more of an impact on us, etc.

There are more rules which determine whether a stimulus is effective or not. These are:

RULE 8

OUR BRAINS LOOK FOR "CRITICAL FEATURES" IN THE ENVIRONMENT. The most critical feature for me at the time was the exit sign. This sign was the one which would give me the cue or information to change direction.

RULE 9

INFORMATION CAN NOT BE PROCESSED INTO THE BRAIN IF IT IS PRESENTED TOO RAPIDLY. I was going too fast to allow the information to be processed by my wife. I needed to slow down so that the information could be processed (effect of speed of presentation).

RULE 10

THE LARGER THE STIMULUS THE EASIER TO PROCESS. The larger the sign, the easier to read (effect of stimulus size).

RULE 11

THE MORE FREQUENTLY THE STIMULUS WAS SHOWN, THE EASIER TO PROCESS. The more frequently the signs were on the roadside, the easier it was to process the information (effect of frequency of presentation).

RULE 12

THE MORE CONTRASTING THE STIMULUS FROM THE BACKGROUND, THE EASIER TO PROCESS. Contrasting, or coloured, or well-lit signs were easier to read (effect of contrast).

RULE 13

THE MORE COMPLEX THE STIMULUS, THE MORE DIFFICULT TO PROCESS. Signs which contained many words and a lot of information were more difficult to read and process. More than one sign placed together made the task even more difficult (effect of complexity).

RULE 14

MULTIPLE STIMULI REDUCED THE ABILITY TO PROCESS. Distractions from my wife, other cars, the landscape, or the sun in my eyes, all reduced the way I could process the information (effect of multiple stimuli).

RULE 15

PROCESSING POWERS ARE REDUCED WITH TIREDNESS. I was fresh in the morning, but as the day wore on I became tired, and had difficulty processing the information from the signs (effect of attention lack).

RULE 16

MOTIVATION INCREASED THE POWERS OF PROCESSING INFORMATION. If I was motivated to leave the freeway at a certain point, I knew I would have to take extra care to read the exit notices, even if this required slowing down and even stopping (the importance of motivation).

RULE 17

ANTICIPATION INCREASED THE POWERS OF PROCESSING. If I could anticipate where the next exit was likely to occur, especially with the use of a map, I was more accurate in the processing of the information (the importance of anticipation).

RULE 18

OVERLOAD OF INFORMATION FROM ANY SOURCE PRODUCED STRESS. If there was too much information provided to my eyes, ears, touch, etc., at any one time, stress occurred and my ability to process the information was reduced (the effect of overload of information).

All these rules are familiar to you in your everyday life. You apply them to your environment automatically, without even thinking about or considering them. The people who know most about them are probably advertising firms and their employees. They wish to attract your attention and then provide information to you which will be of benefit to them (and hopefully, to you).

CHAPTER 14

MORE ON HOW THE BRAIN WORKS

What I have discussed in the previous chapter is the input of *bits* of information into our brain and the conditions in which our brains can best pick up this information; in other words, what catches our eye, or ear, or touch, or taste, or smell.

How the brain deals with this information is still a matter of conjecture, which has been of great interest to many researchers. Professor Luria's ideas, on what he calls functional systems, are easy to understand. He has laid out a plan for us to understand the way in which the information coming in, and going out, is organised. He has spoken in terms of development of functional systems.

Briefly, functional systems may be developed by

1. the individual detecting change from the *status quo* by the use of his sense organs: that is, receiving a "bit" of information;

2. joining this bit of information in the brain with another piece to form a "data base";

3. collecting a group of data bases together to form a "frame of reference";

4. joining frames of reference together to form a single "simple functional system";

5. uniting simple functional systems together to form "complex functional systems": that is, a series of standing orders which allows the individual to function in the environment;

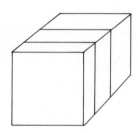

6. uniting complex functional systems together in a variable state as required to fulfill the needs of the person.

When change occurs in the environment, it may be incorporated into the functional systems (assimilation) if the change is slight.

If the change in the environment is great, the functional systems may be modified and a new functional system originated (accommodation).

Because our brain appears to be genetically programmed, or preorganised to work in certain ways as we develop our skill (see Chapter 15, Canalization), we have the meshing together of the genetic preorganisation and the environment. It is by this dynamic process that human growth and development occurs, and this interaction produces what Luria (*The Working Brain*, Penguin Books 1973) calls Complex Functional Systems of the brain.

Unlike the very fixed ideas of many people, who believe there are very specific areas of the brain which do specific tasks and which are the sole providers of that precise function, Luria sees brain functions as having links in many different areas of the brain, both in a vertical and horizontal direction, and says brain function cannot be totally localized to any specific area or isolated cell groups. He says:

... complex functional systems cannot be localized in narrow zones of the cortex or in isolated cell groups, but must be organised in systems of concertedly working zones, each of which performs its role in complex functional systems and which may be located in completely different, and often far distant areas of the brain.

Everything we do depends upon having adequate functional systems, for these systems form the organisational framework in which:

- all sensory input is incorporated,
- all thought is produced,
- all motor activity is directed.

For those who have studied child development, the concept is similar to that attributed to the great French developmentalist, Professor Jean Piaget, who spoke in terms of "schema".

Since the only way information can be received by the brain from the external environment is through the senses (visual, auditory, tactile, taste and smell), to have the correct functional systems it is essential to have correct channels of sensation.

Since the only way information can be sent from the brain to the external environment is through motor function, to have the correct functional systems it is essential to have adequate muscle movement.

In between this sensory input and the motor output is what Nauta and Feitag call the "great intermediate net" (The Brain. *Scientific American*, "The Organisation of the Brain", 1979).

Nauta and Feitag refer to this great intermediate net as "the barrier of intermediate neurones (nerve cells) that interposes itself between the sensory neurones and the motor neurones".

Innumerable functional systems relating to both self-preservation and reproduction occur in both animals and humans. The purpose of these functional systems are, to use a quotation from Fishbein (*Evolution, Development and Children's Learning*, Goodyear, 1976), " . . . in the short term to allow the human to act effectively in the environment, and, in the long term to ensure the survival of the human race."

Those functional systems which appear to be unique to humans, or the most highly developed in humans (given the correct environment), are:

Those relating to sensory abilities —

- Visual: The ability to read the written word.
- Auditory: The ability to hear and understand language.
- Tactile: The ability to finely discriminate by touch.

Those relating to central processing abilities of a high order of integration —

- Perception.
- Memory.
- Thought, etc.

Those relating to motor abilities —

- Walking upright with arms free.
- Talking.
- Manual competence.

Luria also regards each behavioural process (each action), as based on a plan or programme which is aimed for a definite objective. He writes: "Modern

145

psychological investigations have made it clear that each behavioural process is a complex functional system based on a plan, or program of operations, that leads to a definite goal."

Luria uses the body systems as parallel examples with the brain. He regards the digestive system as a complex functional system with many separate parts working towards the objective of digestion. It is the same with the respiratory system or the circulation. Each is made up of a group of functions in different parts of the body, which, working together, attains the selected goal.

The brain is no different. When I wish to type a sentence, I decide the words to type, carry out the motor action required by moving the muscles of my arm and hand, observe the sentence appear on the paper, and compare it with what I had intended. If I see a mistake, the process continues while I correct that mistake. The whole of this intention, action, feedback of information and correction could be classed as a complex functional system.

While we need our higher functions of the brain to decide and plan our aim or goal, much of the rest of the complex functional system is carried out by many different areas of the brain and by other parts of the body.

The development of functional systems takes time and effort. The potential number of functional systems which we each could develop is myriad, and each of us has become selective in what functional systems we develop. While I might like to play tennis and basketball, if I choose to spend the time and energy on playing tennis, I will develop functional systems related to tennis-playing. If I do not, therefore, spend the time and energy on playing basketball, I do not develop functional systems in playing basketball. It is unlikely that my tennis functional systems will be as good as those all-time greats of tennis like Billy Jean King, Margaret Court, Yvonne Goolagong, Hoad, Rosewall, Laver, Newcombe, Connors, Borg, Lendl, McEnroe, etc., who have honed their functional systems to allow them to be the world's best. But I still have functional systems which allow me to play the game, at a greatly reduced standard from them admittedly. We must make a choice of which functional systems to have.

Failure to develop functional systems is seen in the case of the child who is kept locked in a room and makes no contact with a wide environment. This situation is really a state of environmental sensory deprivation and deprivation, of sensation will abort the formation of functional systems.

Similarly, the person who is brain-injured may have, at the time of the injury, lost innumerable functional systems. If he or she is not placed in an environment which is conducive to these functional systems being restored as much as possible, they will be unable to return to function adequately in the environment.

The organisation of the brain

One of the greatest helps to our understanding of the way our brain functions has been the idea that the brain is a hierarchy which works in layers, each with its different function, one on top of the other, with tremendous links between each layer. Some of the great names in medicine and the neural sciences have subscribed to this view. According to Edward Le Winn (*Human Neurological Organisation*,

Charles C. Thomas, 1969), pioneers such as Meynert, Hughlings Jackson, Denny Brown, Doman-Delacato, Bronson and Altman, have all considered the hierarchy of the brain.

One person who has conceived this hierarchy in a behavioural context is Dr Paul MacLean, the Chief of Brain Evolution and Behaviour in The National Institute of Health in the U.S.A. In 1972 he published a paper entitled "The Triune Concept of the Brain". His approach has been summarized by Professor Carl Sagan in his book *The Dragons of Eden* (Random House, 1977). Sagan quotes Maclean, "We are obliged to look at ourselves and the world through the eyes of three different mentalities," two of which lack the power of speech. The human brain, MacLean holds, "amounts to three interconnected biological computers, each with its own special sense of time and space, its own memory, motor and other functions."

MacLean, along with the other researchers, theorized that each brain layer has a *sensory input* and a *motor output* which is peculiar to that level, and which is dependent upon the lower layers functioning adequately.

Basically, it may be that there are four layers to the brain, placed one on top of the other:

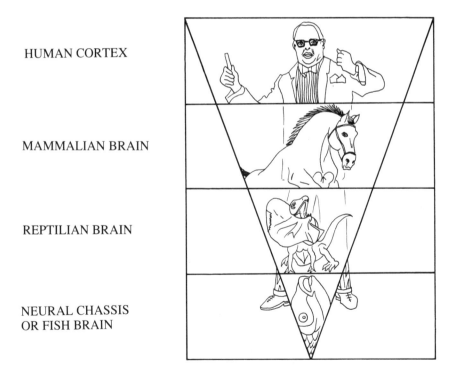

HUMAN CORTEX

MAMMALIAN BRAIN

REPTILIAN BRAIN

NEURAL CHASSIS
OR FISH BRAIN

Fig. 14.1. The four layers of the brain.

THE NEURAL CHASSIS OR FISH BRAIN

The lowest layer of the brain is the most primitive and is found in fishes. It really consists of the brainstem, which controls the so-called "vegetable functions" of respiration, blood pressure, etc. This has been called the neural "chassis", and it is the chassis on which the rest of the brain is built. The arousal centre, the reticular formation, runs through the middle of this brainstem.

Sensory input through visual, vestibular (or our balance mechanisms) and touch mechanisms occur, and motor output consists of movement of the head, the body, and the front and back limbs. This is similar to a baby who moves the limbs and wriggles the body, but can make no definite forward movement.

THE REPTILIAN BRAIN

On top of the neural chassis is the next layer of the brain. It, plus the neural chassis, is known as the reptilian brain. This reptile layer depends upon correct function of the neural chassis and cannot exist by itself. According to Maclean there are certain behaviours which are more strongly developed at this brain level than in the neural chassis. These he identifies as a very strong territorial control urge, a hierarchy of power in the form of a pecking order, a strong sense of ritual and an aggressive stance on these matters. It has been said that the place to see these qualities in their most obvious form in the human is to attend a parliamentary session.

Motor output in this brain produces a forward movement with the abdomen or belly downwards and with the limbs moving in a pattern, one front and one back limb working together on the same side of the body, while supporting the body weight, much like a crocodile.

THE MAMMALIAN BRAIN

When another brain layer is placed above the reptilian brain, it is dependent on both the reptilian brain and the neural chassis. This becomes the mammalian brain. This additional layer consists of a specific area in the brain which is known as the limbic system. In this limbic system is developed the emotional brain, which gives to mammals the ability to love and to empathize with others (that is, the ability to feel for, and care about, others). Thus mammals, such as dogs, horses, dolphins, etc., have the ability to relate to others, beside their own family, in a caring way.

Probably at this level also is a strong concept of reciprocal obligations, which is the ability to join together for the good of the species, so that the species will survive: to search together for food, to bind together in defence — the concept that in unity is strength.

One story which demonstrates this reciprocal obligation in a very dramatic way, concerns a Korean warrior who died and who was taken to hell to observe what occurred there. He saw tables laden with food, with great delicacies. The eating utensils provided were chopsticks. He saw that they were about two metres long and no person was able to reach his mouth with the food at the end of the chopstick. When he observed the people, he saw them to be separated from each other, looking intensely miserable and underfed. He asked to be taken back to heaven and upon entering saw the same food on the tables but the people were gathered in groups, happy and using the chopsticks to feed each other. Those in hell had obviously remained in their reptilian brain; those in heaven were in their mammalian brain.

Motor output at this level sees a change in the pattern of movement, a cross pattern, with the legs diagonally opposite each other moving together. The right front leg will move with the left back leg and vice versa.

THE HUMAN CORTEX

Above the mammalian brain and incorporating all the functions of the other three brains is the human cortex. Not only does it use the functions of the other brains, it has also developed special qualities of its own. We anticipate, we initiate, we explore. As Richard Leakey puts it in his book, *The Making of Mankind* (Michael Joseph, 1981), "No other animal manipulates the world in the extensive and arbitrary way that humans do."

We have developed fine powers of DISCRIMINATION. It is upon this ability that we have built our civilization. This discrimination is both sensory and motor.

Sensory Discrimination

We have immense powers to pick up the sensation of seeing and hearing and touch. If we find that our power of discrimination is inadequate, we enlarge those powers by new initiatives and explorations. What we constantly do is to make the stimuli more effective by enlarging the stimuli, or improving our abilities to detect stimuli by artificial means. Briefly, we can easily think of ways in which we have achieved this.

Visually, we are not limited by our naked eye. Because we wish to see in the distance, we have developed telescopes. Because we wish to see objects smaller than is possible with the naked eye, we have developed microscopes.

In sound, we have developed from the primitive loudspeaker to enormous broadcast systems to send out our messages, and conversely we have developed machines that will pick up sounds that our naked ears could not possibly hear.

In our touch sensation, we have shifted threat away from our own intimate and personal space, first of all by the use of primitive weapons, such as shields and basic missiles, then by fortification of a specific encampment or fort. Now we have moved past these close personal body areas to the concept of star wars in outer space.

Motor Discrimination

Our brain's motor functions have kept pace with our sensory abilities.

The way we can manipulate tools lies in the power of the thumb and fingers working together. From the first grasp and use of a stone or a stick have come an expanding capacity to develop great earthmoving tools which we can control with our fingers and with which can move mountains.

We have also moved into an erect position, off our abdomen or belly-down position, and can walk upright (with our arms initially used for balance). Now we have freed the arms from the primary balance role, and use them at the same time as we move our legs and bodies. Our mobility has grown from slowly moving ourselves on our own legs on land to rapid transit on land, on water, under the water and in the air by the use of our exploration and creative initiatives. (If you refer to the development of the human infant, you will note that to obtain this upright stance, the infant goes through the fish stage, the reptilian stage and the mammalian stage as she or he develops strength and co-ordination of motor output.)

What binds all of these things together is language: our ability to understand and to express words, and the other symbolic languages we use. Without language, little of the major explorations of our world would have been possible. Without language few of our reciprocal obligations could have been fulfilled, and little of this creative exploration would have been accomplished.

The cortex is responsible for all these marvellous acts and developments of vision, sound, touch, hand function, mobility, language. No other animal is like us, for we carry within us, and are dependent upon, all of those three brains which sit below our cortex. Without them we would have no base on which to function.

Almost nothing gets to our cortex without going through these other three brains. Virtually nothing gets out of our cortex without going through these three brains. And in both, the entry and the exit pathways, enormous modifications of both sensory inputs and motor outputs occur.

THE POLICYMAKERS — THE EXECUTIVE — THE WORKERS

Perhaps the easiest way to see how brain organisation works is to examine the functions which are common to all human endeavour, whether in one person or in a major organisation.

POLICYMAKERS

THE EXECUTIVE

THE WORKERS

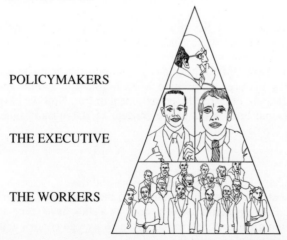

Fig. 14.2. The function of an organisation

150

Every organisation works on three important levels, which are interdependent. These three levels consist of:

firstly, those who make the policies;

secondly, the executive, which is responsible for ensuring that the work is correctly organised and performed at the "coalface" by the workers;

thirdly, the workers, who actually do the work.

A. The Brain Policy Makers

The brain, which organises our being in the world, works on the same principles. In general, the policymakers are in contact with the executive, but are isolated from the workers. In the same way the cortex is in touch with the executive, but isolated from the workers. The part of the brain appearing to be most involved with policy are the frontal lobes.

This isolation of our cortex from the world is essential, if we are to function properly. Our cortex is responsible for the big decisions in life. It is concerned with policy matters.

On the input side of the cortex, the brain would never be able to take the load of information coming in through all the senses without that information being thoroughly screened, sifted and given priority. Imagine the President of the United States being inundated with the problems of 250 million Americans. There would be a massive overload, and the President would not be able to function in a policymaking role.

The output side presents the same problem. Just as the President would be totally incapable of personally providing all the services done in his name, so is the cortex totally incapable of personally undertaking all the motor activities of hand function, movement of body and limbs, and speech.

The cortex is totally dependent upon the other three brains to work correctly. These other three brains have to screen out unimportant stimuli, information and messages, select the things which are important and allocate priorities of attention for the cortex to deal with. This is the same as the Head of Government. The only matters which gain his attention are those which are most important. For him to do otherwise leads to overload and to disaster.

What the President does, like all organisations, whether it is a hospital, a military base, a factory or a corporate organisation, is to have an executive. The Government makes the policy and hands it on to the executive whose work is to see that the policy is carried out. The policymakers of the brain function in exactly the same manner as the policymakers of government. They anticipate, initiate, consider consequences of their actions, co-ordinate activities with other similar beings, in an attempt to ensure survival.

B. The Executive

The work of the executive is to assess all information coming from the work place, deal with those matters which it is competent to undertake, prepare a priority listing for the policymakers, and present it in a manageable form to them (that is, up the chain of command). The decisions of the policymakers are then given to the executive, which transforms the policy into action through the workers (that is, down the chain of command). If the executive is not functioning correctly, wrong information or wrong priority allocations will be given to the policymakers, or incorrect instructions will be given to the workers, and the organisation will cease to function properly.

C. Workers

There are two major groups of workers. There are those who collect the information, and in the body we call them the sensors. Through touch, vision, hearing, taste, smell, balance and muscle position they constantly feed information up the chain of command to the executive: into the lower ranks first, where it is allocated a priority rating before being directed further up the hierarchical chain, if necessary. Failure of any of the sensors means that inadequate information will be presented to the executive. If this occurs, it is possible that different sensors will be used, or else decisions made by the executive will be based on incorrect or inadequate information. This leads to incorrect policy.

The second group of workers are those which are the motor workers. This is the action group. It consists of all the muscles in the body, plus the nerves which feed directly to them and control them. These workers provide all motor power. If the nerve or the muscle is damaged, the work will not be done correctly; this lack of output or incorrect output will become obvious, and will be notified back up the chain of command to the management or executive level, where action will be taken to use other muscle workers. If failure of output is still apparent, this information would be fed back to the policymakers, who would determine whether to vary the work by altering the programme, or cease attempting to reach the objective.

RULE 19

THE BRAIN IS A HIERARCHICAL ORGAN. IT HAS FOUR MAJOR LAYERS.

RULE 20

BRAIN FUNCTION IS RESTORED FROM THE BASE UPWARD.

RULE 21

ANY BREAK IN THE CHAIN OF COMMAND, UP OR DOWN THE NERVOUS SYSTEM, WILL CHANGE THE ABILITY OF THE PERSON TO FUNCTION.

RULE 22

THE NERVOUS SYSTEM WILL SUBSTITUTE OTHER NON-DAMAGED PARTS OF THE SYSTEM IN AN ATTEMPT TO COMPENSATE FOR THE DAMAGED PARTS.

WHAT YOU REALLY WANT IN THE SEVERELY BRAIN INJURED IS THE RESTORATION OF FUNCTIONAL SYSTEMS.

IT IS IMPORTANT WITH ALL PATIENTS TO BE AWARE OF THESE RULES, AND TO APPLY THEM TO ALL CASES TO THE THERAPY WHICH NEEDS TO BE GIVEN.

CHAPTER 15

THE PATHWAY OF RECOVERY

Life is dynamic. Even when a person has been severely injured, as long as they survive, the dynamic processes of the body continue. Repair is what we call this dynamic process following injury. If you have a cut on your skin, repair commences almost immediately. If you have a stomach ulcer, as long as the factors which brought it about are ceased or reduced, the process of repair can commence.

Nature is very conservation conscious. There is always a fixed pattern for repair, which is followed in almost all cases, but which is modified slightly depending upon the tissue involved. These patterns of repair occur, because they make the most efficient use of the resources of the body. If the tissue can be replaced by the same type of tissue as was damaged, this is the best method. This is most easily seen following sunburn, when the damaged skin peels off and is replaced by new skin. Where the damage is excessive, such as a deep burn, new skin may not be replaced, and instead scar tissue or fibrous tissue is formed.

In the brain, while it is accepted that *repair* of damaged brain cells does take place, it is also considered that *replacement* of dead brain cells does not occur. While this statement is currently being disputed, it is best for you to remain with the old thinking and consider that dead brain cells are not replaced. If you do this, you will not be seen as argumentative by the health professions.

What you do have to consider is that you have three major concepts with which you must become familiar. These concepts are the basis of your work with the patient.

It is best to call this set the TRIAD.

This triad consists of:

1. the concept of CANALIZATION;
2. the concept of SPARE CAPACITY;
3. the concept of NEUROLOGICAL (BRAIN) RE-ORGANISATION.

The concept of CANALIZATION will be dealt with here. The other two concepts will be dealt with in a future book. Each is very important for your knowledge and consideration. Each is vital to the recovery of function of your patient. Each is still disputed by many in the health-care professions. Each is easily recognizable as logical to the normal person.

The concept of Canalization

At the University of Cincinnati, Fishbein (*Evolution, Development and Children's Learning*, Goodyear Developmental Psychology Series, Goodyear Publishing Company, California, 1976) uses the term coined by Waddington in 1960 of — "Canalization".

Canalization refers to the *universal drive* in a *prearranged direction* as children develop from infancy to adulthood, and into the different stages of adulthood until death. Waddington believed that canalization involves "a set of genetic processes which ensure that development will proceed in the normal ways", and that "more and more evidence suggests that human behaviour has a high degree of preorganisation, which causes the paths human learning can take to be constrained. The human being is designed to organise in certain ways as he grows."

Fishbein considers that this canalization works throughout the lifetime of the individual.

If you are familiar with the work of the great developmentalists such as Jean Piaget, Gesell, Erickson, etc., you will be aware that common to these teachers is the idea that all children pass through stages of growth which are in a correct sequence. This sequence is frequently viewed as fixed and unchangeable. All children pass through the stages in the same order. As an example of the sequence in the development of motor function, children learn to move and then to crawl and then to creep on all fours and then to stand hanging onto the furniture and then to cruise from one piece of furniture to another and then to walk without support.

Shakespeare said the same thing in regard to the seven ages of man in *As You Like It*. He wrote

"All the world's a stage,
And all the men and women merely players:
They have their exits and their entrances;
And one man in his time plays many parts,
His acts being seven ages. At first the infant,
Mewling and puking in his nurse's arms . . . "

He was saying that there is a sequence of life, fixed and unchangeable, which goes through the lifetime of the individual. Tied in with the direction of this pathway is the fact that there must be an intrinsic drive within each person which pushes them along the pathway.

Professor White, Professor of Psychology at Harvard University, in his Foreword to Fishbein's book writes that "Humans have inbuilt constructive capacities — that all tend towards predictable channels of development and organisation."

It is very likely that this canalization process, or these inbuilt constructive capacities, are controlled by the genetic makeup of the individual, and the drive along a fixed pathway is as much present in the person who is brain-injured as it is in the person who is not brain-injured.

There are two important aspects of canalization which need consideration. They

155

are the *Intrinsic Drive* which is built into all of us, and the *Fixed Pathway* along which this drive takes us.

The Intrinsic Drive

No one would seriously dispute that the most basic drives relate to self-preservation and reproduction. These drives are immensely strong and designed to ensure the survival of the individual and of the species.

Self-preservation is familiar to us. We would not have survived to the age where we can read this book without having a strong desire for self-preservation. We all know that to preserve ourselves, we need to be able to detect a threat to our existence and to be able to deal with it. Those who are involved in military service or the police are better trained in methods of ensuring survival under hazardous conditions, but we all depend on the ability to fight or flee or accommodate in our reactions to changes in our environment, especially if they are dangerous.

Under normal conditions, when we are functioning well, living, working, playing as we wish, we are able to deal with danger, unless it moves outside our experience. When we fall sick or are injured, our abilities to fight or to flee or to negotiate a settlement favourable to us are decreased. We are handicapped and an intense drive comes into us to regain health.

This drive to recover from ill-health is familiar to all of us who, having been sick, earnestly desire to start to eat, to use our sight and our hearing and our touch, to move our bodies and limbs, to get out of bed and walk and to gain control of our bowels and bladder. There is no scientific evidence of which I know which demonstrates that this desire is lost in the brain-injured person. Quite to the contrary, my experience has shown that even the most severely brain-injured patient has an innate desire, and desperately wants, to become well.

In my work I am constantly asked to see patients who are regarded by their doctors as being "vegetative": having no ability to relate to people or to the environment. Almost without exception, these patients have been able to demonstrate that they have thoughts and desires which they can communicate by facial expression and by other body language. Certainly the way in which they do this is terribly limited, but the fact that they do communicate is important.

The very fact that these patients have not curled up into a ball and refused to interact with people implies that they are motivated to remain in contact with life, even if their abilities to do so are minimal.

As the brain-injured person regains function, the evidence of motivation becomes stronger. As they become aggressive, it becomes more apparent still. This is all evidence of the seeking for independence, of the drive which is in all of us to gain control of our environment.

If we, who are the significant people in the environment, block their efforts constantly and prevent this drive from being productive, the patient, seeing that winning is not going to be allowed by the health system, after a prolonged period of time may sink into apathy and may die. Even with the patient sunk in apathy, I have seen the desire to survive rekindled and flame, when the correct environment or surroundings are provided.

One of the most necessary things needed for drive to flow is love, especially from the family. Concern from all health carers is also of great importance. A book which gives the essentials of this is by Dr Gerald Jampolsky, *Teach Only Love*, (Bantam Books, 1983).

Tied in with love is hope. As Professor Kutscher of Columbia Presbyterian Medical Center has written, "Hope must be an active force in every life, always offering a promise of fulfillment, involvement with living, and an expansion of life's horizons." (*Hope: the Dynamics of Self Fulfillment*, Arnold Hutschnecker, G.P. Putnam, New York, 1981.)

The Fixed Pathway

Many workers have seen the parallel between the development of the infant to adulthood and the recovery of the brain-injured patient from the effects of their trauma. In children this has been commented upon by people such as Dr Glenn Doman at the Institute for the Achievement of Human Potential in Philadelphia, U.S.A., who is the Director of Research at that Institute, Dr E. Lewinn, Dr Carl Delacato and Dr Ayres of the U.S.A.

In working with stroke victims, some researchers have also expressed this view. Dr T.E. Twitchell in 1951 ("The Restoration of Motor Function in Man", *Brain.*, 74.) made the statement following his observations of stroke patients that

"The restoration of motor function . . . followed a general pattern in which certain phenomena predominated during distinct phases or stages of recovery. It soon became clear that the evolution of recovery of those patients in whom restoration of motor function was not complete also followed the same general pattern."

In his work observing patients for one year, following coma of at least two weeks' duration, Dr A. Bricolo and his colleagues of Verona, Italy (*Journal of Neurosurgery*, 1980, 52. 625-634) saw that prolonged coma was a dynamic condition moving increasingly towards the regaining of complex brain function. He saw definite milestones in the return of vigilance, return of the ability to obey commands and, lastly, speech, setting a pattern of recovery. He did not see all things occur in all patients under his care. A significant number failed to progress to a point of good recovery. He was, however, able to see a definite pattern which could be considered the process of canalization in action in the severely brain-injured.

It is worth consideration that the "fixed pathway" described by Piaget, Kagan and others in the child, the process of "canalization" described by Waddington, the "general pattern" described by Twitchell and the pathway of recovery of Bricolo are the same process, but seen at different ages or under different conditions.

In a practical setting this has been confirmed in work with patients studied during the time of their coma and provided with the coma arousal programme. This pattern of recovery has been quite definite. The beauty of such a pattern is that it can be used as a map upon which the position of the patient can be determined, and along which the course of his recovery can be plotted. You will recall how I wrote in the Introduction about the necessity of having a guide and a map. The

157

questionnaire in Chapter 9, "The Questionnaire to Find Out the State of the Patient", is the basis on which we plot the position of the patient. It also shows the way forward.

The Glasgow Coma Scale provided in some detail in Chapter 2, "Measuring the Patient's Condition and What It Means", can be seen as a scale which looks for basic milestones in the patient who is brain-injured and in coma. As the patient comes out of the coma, they follow a definite pathway of recovery which can be measured. Ascending as they do along this fixed pathway, they gain more points on the coma scale.

Let us have a look at the different brain levels which are involved as a person goes into, or comes out of, coma. Usually the person who goes into coma from brain injury does so immediately following the accident. Some, however, who have a so-called lucid interval, may get up following the accident, walk around and talk for a period of minutes or even hours before going into coma. These patients go through a pattern of loss of speech and other motor actions until they go into coma. They have a progressive loss of their brain function, which can be easily detected by any observer.

Most people will not be familiar with the picture of a severely brain-injured patient with a lucid interval. One similar process which produces coma without such dire consequences is familiar to us all either by observation or experience. I was at a lecture given by Mr Art Sandler and Ms Sandy Brown of Philadelphia. U.S.A., two consultants on brain injury, in 1981, where they used the example of the effect of alcohol on brain function and the pathway which slowly unfolds as the conscious, aware person steadily drinks his way into coma.

While this means, for our understanding, that we are "backing" our way into coma, it does allow us to link coma into a phenomenon which is familiar to us.

A person who is aware, wide-awake, fully conscious, undergoes certain changes which can be observed quite readily when they commence to drink alcohol. Before they start drinking, their sensory abilities are working, allowing them to pick up many aspects of their environment. They are able to look and see what is going on around them, will hear any conversation directed at them and will comprehend its meaning. They will be able to feel a coin placed in their hand and be able to tell which side is heads and which is tails. They will be able to smell perfumes and will be able to taste their food.

Their motor abilities are also working well. They will be able to stand up straight, and if asked to move, will shift their body in the correct direction in a balanced manner until they reach their target. If asked to pick up a pin from the table, they will reach out their hand and, using thumb and index finger, will grasp the pin and place it where directed. When they are engaged in conversation, they will speak, and words will come out with the correct words in the correct order with the correct amount of power.

Their first drink or two may not have a great deal of effect on them, but as they continue to drink more the brain becomes less able to function correctly. If they continue to drink, they may eventually be "dead drunk", lying on the floor semi-comatose or even in coma.

During their passage down to coma they go through a broad pattern which can be identified. They lose brain and body function in a set pattern. On their way back they also come through certain stages which we can identify and which can be used to illustrate the pathway of recovery of the patient from coma. The patient coming out of coma from severe brain injury, however, is moving a great deal more slowly. There are seven stages which can be used. These are:

Stage Seven	The Stage of Creativity
Stage Six	The Stage of Fine Discrimination
Stage Five	The Stage of Coarse Discrimination
Stage Four	The Stage of Localization
Stage Three	The Stage of Localized Withdrawal
Stage Two	The Stage of Reflex Generalized Withdrawal
Stage One	The Stage of No Response

Stage Seven — The Stage of Creativity

If we look at our person before going into the pathway leading to coma, they start at Stage Seven. At this stage they are fully conscious and able to use their brain in a creative way. If the person is a musician or a poet they will be able to compose and create. They can pay attention to their environment and direct their brain to any problems in hand. Their memory is good.

Stage Six — The Stage of Fine Discrimination

Our drinker starts to lose powers of fine discrimination. Sensory abilities start to decrease. Vision may not now be as good. When looking at the menu, he or she may now need to move it closer to their eyes or even put on glasses. Hearing may not be as acute. The person may not comprehend as normally as before. Touch may not be as sensitive. He or she may have lost the ability to detect which side of the coin is handed to them. They may also have lost their fine sense of taste and smell.

There are now some slight difficulties with attention. He or she finds concentrating on a specific matter more difficult. Their memory may not be as good as normal, and they have some difficulty working out problems which before were easy to them. They are more likely to put them aside if they are too hard.

Motor abilities are also slightly decreased. He or she has lost their "edge". Their movements are not quite as controlled. When they stand, balance and force of movement and direction may need some slight correction. When reaching out to pick up the pin between thumb and index finger, they may fumble and need more than one attempt. Speech is also slightly decreased in quality. They will tend to use a smaller vocabulary and may also repeat some words.

Since vision and hearing and touch and attention span and memory and balance and hand function and speech are not quite as good as before, he or she will find that they are not able to do things as easily. This may be of no concern to them, but if they do want to perform some motor action and they cannot, they may become frustrated and a trifle irritable.

Stage Five — The Stage of Coarse Discrimination

As our drinker continues to drink, more of the brain becomes affected. Sensory abilities are now decreasing considerably. This means that he or she may have trouble processing the information which is in their environment. They now have to stare wide-eyed at things which they wish to look at, and it takes longer to see what they are. They may also find it hard to hear what is being said to them and may ask for it to be repeated. Touch abilities are decreased, and he or she has trouble feeling objects with their hands. Comprehension or understanding of words whether spoken or written becomes increasingly poor.

Attention span is now very short, and he or she has trouble concentrating on anything for other than a brief period of time. They are easily deflected from any task. Memory often appears to be out of control and provides them with information which may not be relevant to the environment in which they find themselves. Their powers of thinking are greatly diminished.

Motor abilities are greatly reduced. He or she has trouble standing up and may stagger. Their balance mechanisms are affected, and they are unable to walk a straight line. When they reach out to pick up their next glass of alcohol, the movement is unco-ordinated and they may knock the glass over. When they do attempt to take something in their hand, they use the palm of their hand to grasp it rather than finger and thumb. Speech is now poorly controlled, with the wrong words coming out. He or she finds that they are not able to be understood. When the words do come, they are often in an incorrect sequence.

Our drinker's emotional state now becomes more inappropriate. Because he or she now cannot perform the motor actions they require, they are at the mercy of their environment. They become frustrated and may even become aggressive, attempting to fight everybody, apart from those who are especially known to them. Or else, he or she becomes apathetic and will slide off their chair and into a corner.

Stage Four — The Stage of Localization

As our drinker continues to drink, his or her understanding of the spoken word, apart from very familiar sentences or phrases, disappears. They lose their ability to localize. They may have difficulty moving their eyes to their glass of beer, and in detecting the position of objects or people they wish to see. They become disorientated in time and place and with people. They look like they are lost in their environment.

Their attention span is almost non-existent. They tend to wish to sleep, but may waken with a start. If you asked him or her to look into your eyes, they would be unable to do so. There is no evidence that they have memory and they may not even react greatly with those who are very familiar to them.

Motor abilities are now greatly decreased. He or she cannot move themselves from place to place, except with the greatest difficulty. Their body is unstable, and they may have difficulty even creeping on their hands and knees along the floor. They may sag from side to side, fall and get back into the creep position. Hand function is now very primitive, and while he or she still may be able to grasp with their hands, the grasp is very much by palm and fingers, and they are unable to bring finger and thumb together. Speech, apart from a few emotional swear-words, has virtually disappeared.

Stage Three — The Stage of Localized Withdrawal

Our drinker has lost almost all evidence of awareness of his or her environment. Use of eyes and ears has virtually disappeared, as far as an observer can judge. This may not be the case, however, and a loud noise may startle them. If they are hurt on the arm by the application of pain, they may withdraw the limb and moan.

He or she appears to be asleep (possibly with heavy breathing), often has lost control of the bladder, may lose saliva from the mouth (producing a heavy dribble). He or she cannot now swallow.

Motor function has almost totally disappeared. He or she now lies where they have fallen, lying on their side, back or front. They may make some spontaneous or random movements with their arms or legs, but they will be very weak and unco-ordinated and apparently without purpose. Hand function is very poor. They have let go of the bottle because the hand opens and cannot grasp it. There is no speech, although he or she may still make some noise if disturbed forcefully.

Stage Two — The Stage of Reflex Generalized Withdrawal

Normal noises or touching brings no response. He is "out like a light". A very heavy or painful touch or intense noise may bring a start where he may move his whole body or it may just bring a flicker of the eyelid. Movement is virtually non-existent.

Stage One — The Stage of No Response

This may be almost a pre-death stage. Evidence of life is determined not by the actions of the drinker which are nil, but by close observation of breathing, heart rate, blood pressure, pupil size and reaction: that is, brainstem function.

What we have observed has been the progressive loss of cortical (higher brain) function, until only subcortical and eventually a similar brainstem function remain. It would be incorrect to consider that each of these stages listed above was a watertight compartment. Different people lose function at different levels, but the analogy is worth consideration.

The Recovery Process

When recovery occurs, we see a restoring of the lost function following a similar pathway. First of all, sensory abilities, especially pain sensation and then hearing, begin to recover, then evidence of sight. Initially, all these things are still in a very primitive stage. Movement may be almost non-existent, or only on a reflex basis. This reflex basis may produce a generalized body response to any stimulus, and then move on to a localized arm or leg response. Then the ability to localize stimuli by touch, hearing or vision may return. Motor function, such as moving the head, arms, legs, body, etc., may at first be random, but slowly may come back to a controlled movement. Thought and memory function also return, unless permanent damage has been done.

While this restoration of function occurs relatively rapidly from the alcoholic state, recovery from coma and severe brain injury may be greatly prolonged, and, depending upon the extent of the brain injury, may not be fully accomplished. How far along the Fixed Pathway the patient will travel will depend upon factors dealt with in Chapter 4.

CHAPTER 16

THE SPARE CAPACITY OF THE BRAIN

Although we all safeguard our close personal space, if we only had that area in which to live we would feel very restricted. We like to have room to move. Our thinking demands that we are able to go out of what we normally use, if we need to, into additional areas which we may use only occasionally. That is why we go on holidays or to the beach or into the bush.

When we build a house, we always allow for extra space in each room. We do not cramp ourselves into the very minimum space in our bathroom or bedroom or kitchen; we leave room to move.

When we build a sports stadium or an opera house, we do not build for the usual number of people who might attend a function; we always build enough spare space to take a capacity crowd. When a road is built, it is never built just to carry the average number of vehicles; it always has the capacity to carry more than the usual traffic. If our house or our stadiums or our entertainment areas or our roads begin to use up that spare capacity which is built in, we become concerned, see the lack of spare capacity as a problem, and seek to provide more, so that we constantly have a capacity to spare.

While the speed limit may be 50 mph or 60 kph, few people would be satisfied with a vehicle which could only reach that speed. We like to have spare engine capacity, which we can use if we run into trouble. Although many cars carry only the driver for most of the time, cars without room for passengers are not popular.

This demand for spare capacity in our environment is a reflection of the way in which our brains, and all parts of our body, function.

With our leg muscles, while we could exist in our civilization, in general, if we merely walked, we like to have the capacity to run if we wish to, both for enjoyment and as a safeguard for our approach distance.

With our organs, we know that there is a tremendous spare capacity. If one eye is damaged, we still use the other. If one ear is damaged, we still use the other. If one kidney or lung or a substantial part of the bowel is removed, we know that there is a spare capacity. All the transplantation programmes that have been devised have been to restore capacity of the organ.

Even our reproductive systems have an enormous spare capacity. The number of ova which a female liberates from the ovaries and which have the potential to be fertilized, given the correct conditions, is enormous. The number of sperm manufactured, and ejected at emission, runs into hundreds of thousands per cubic centimetre of seminal fluid, yet only one sperm usually penetrates the ova.

This spare capacity appears to be a safeguard by nature to ensure

- the survival of the individual
- and also the continuation of the species

and is demonstrated by the spare capacity of organs, such as the kidneys, lungs, liver and bowel in the first instance, and by the excess of the sperm and ova in the second.

The brain appears to be no exception to this rule of spare capacity. When at school we were all told that we use only 10 per cent of our brain. Obviously the teacher thought that we had much more capacity to do the study and work than we were at that time using.

While it is a common belief that most people only utilize a minimal amount of their brain tissue, until recently this has been a difficult assertion to justify.

Work done in this area by Professor John Lorber, Research Professor of Paediatrics at Sheffield University in England, was published in a paper for the journal *Science* (Vol. 210, 12.12.80) entitled "Is Your Brain Really Necessary?" In it he discussed his findings following the C.T. scan (brain X-ray) of 600 patients with hydrocephalus (the so-called water-on-the-brain).

Lorber divided his patients into four categories.

The most severely affected group were those in whom fluid filled 95 per cent of the cranial cavity.

In this group he found:

a. Many were severely disabled. (Note that some were not disabled.)

b. Half of the patients had an I.Q. greater than 100.

c. There was one young man who had an I.Q. of 126 and who had gained First Class Honours in mathematics.

The reviewer of the article says, "What is surprising, however, is that a substantial proportion of patients appear to escape functional impairment in spite of grossly abnormal brain structure." In plain English, the reviewer says that many of the patients could do far more than was expected, considering the lack of brain.

Lorber concluded from his work: "There must be a tremendous amount of redundancy or spare capacity in the brain, just as there is with the kidney and liver", and "The cortex (higher brain) probably is responsible for a great deal less than most people imagine." He raised the question in regard to the student with an I.Q. of 126: "How can someone with a grossly reduced cerebral mantle, not only move among his fellows with no apparent social deficit, but also reach high academic achievement?"

Professor Wall, Professor of Anatomy, University College, London, England, in the same article makes the comment, "For hundreds of years neurologists have assumed that all that is dear to them is performed by the cortex, but it may well be that the deep structures in the brain carry out many of the functions assumed to be the sole province of the cortex."

In correspondence with Professor Lorber in 1981 I suggested that a person with 5 per cent brain working in an organised way may be better off than a person with more brain working in a disorganised way, and that many brain-injured people with even a 90 per cent functioning brain are mentally retarded because of the brain being disorganised rather than having an inadequate amount. I also suggested that the correct way to deal with the problem is to seek to reorganise correctly the disorganised brain. Professor Lorber wrote to me, "I think that your surmises are very largely in accordance with my views."

There were other interesting questions which Professor Lorber's paper also raised, and which challenge very heavily the orthodox thinking in regard to brain function.

In one group of 50 patients with hydrocephalus on one side only, a minority showed what would normally be expected in such patients: that is, the opposite side of the body and limbs with paralysis and spasticity (tight muscles).

Lorber also remarked on one patient who had a spasticity on the same side as his hydrocephalic brain: "This is exactly the opposite to all that we learnt at medical school."

Lorber also commented on the fact that when a shunt to drain away excess fluid from the brain of a young hydrocephalic patient was implanted, complete restoration of overall brain function sometimes occurs. He writes, "There must be some true regeneration of brain substance in some sense, but I'm not necessarily saying that nerve cells regenerate. I don't think anyone knows."

Professor David Bower, Professor of Neurophysiology at Liverpool University, England, says, "Although Lorber's work does not demonstrate that we don't need a brain, it does show that the brain can work in conditions we would have thought impossible."

Other information is also available to us on this topic of spare capacity.

The brain weight of an adult is normally in the range of 1200-1500 gm. The weight of a normal newborn infant's brain is about 350 gm. There are some people with a condition of microcephaly, whose brains never develop to the normal size and may, in fact, remain at much the same size as a newborn infant's brain.

Reports in the world medical literature tell of some patients who are microcephalic, who obviously could perform significant function with a greatly decreased quantity of brain tissue.

Dr Dooling and Dr Richardson of the Neurology-Neuropathology Department of the Massachusetts General Hospital reported on the autopsy findings of a 20-year-old female patient with microcephaly in the *Arch. Neurology*, Vol 37, Nov. 1980.

Instead of the expected brain weight of 1160 gm, the brain weighed 260 gm, the equivalent of the brain weight of an infant of eight months' gestation (that is, one month before birth). Yet this person "learned to walk at three years, said a few words at five years, and was toilet trained in later childhood. She was able to wash, and partly dress herself, ate with a fork and spoon, helped with some household chores, listened to the radio, and attended movies."

These authors also refer to another person, a 48-year-old woman with a brain weight of 370 gm, who was able to walk, say some phrases in French, German and Swiss, and cared for her needs in an institutional setting.

Their conclusions are similar to Lorber's. They write, "How great the discrepancy between the size and functional capacity can be, is shown by the skills our patient mastered with so small a brain."

If a person is brain-injured, the chance of losing massive quantities of brain and surviving must be very rare, if not impossible. While I know of no work which details the *amount* of brain lost in the most severely brain-injured survivors, I would doubt that it could be anywhere in the vicinity even of 20 per cent, which means that there must be at least 80 per cent of brain still remaining.

It would, therefore, seem that we must assume that there is a remarkable spare capacity of the brain, which will lie dormant if not brought into action, but may be "hooked" back into work if a correct approach is made.

The first thing which needs to be changed is the attitude that nothing can be done. Each brain-injured patient who survives should be looked at very closely with the thought in the back of your mind:

THIS PATIENT MUST HAVE ENORMOUS SPARE BRAIN CAPACITY.

This must be followed by the question;

HOW DO WE BRING IT INTO USE?

We know that the only way we can use this spare capacity is to demand that it should be used. Of course, when you start to bring this spare capacity into action, what you are really doing is reorganising the brain. The theory of this will be dealt with in the next chapter of this section and the practical part in the Therapy Section to follow.

CHAPTER 17

THE REORGANISATION OF THE BRAIN

NEUROLOGICAL REORGANISATION   *THE PLASTICITY OF THE BRAIN*

The existence of plasticity is not a point of minor practical significance. If all levels of life are open to change, then there is great reason to be optimistic about the ability of intervention programmes to enhance human development.

Professor Richard Lerner, *On the Nature of Human Plasticity*, (Cambridge University Press, 1984.)

The brain is a constantly changing organ. It is enormously responsive to the environment. Dr Jose Delgado, Chairman of the Department of Physiological Sciences at the Autonomous Medical School in Madrid and Director of Research for the National Centre Ramon y Cajal expresses the importance of the environment in the words, "The brain is a dynamic organ exquisitely responsive to the environment." (*Mind and Supermind*. Ed. Albert Rosenfeld. Holt Rhinehart and Winston, New York, 1977.)

As you read this book, even this chapter, even these words, your brain is changing. As your brain takes in information, it must check it against your memory and decide what to do with it. New information presents itself to you as an interruption or change from the pattern you already know. It is when there is a discrepancy between old knowledge and new information that you register change — and learn.

Nothing occurs in isolation. When learning takes place there must be changes which occur in the cells in the brain. Just as the poet John Donne wrote many years ago, "No man (or woman) is an Island, entire of itself, every man is a piece of the Continent a part of the Maine", so is every cell. No cell works in isolation. It is always linked in with a myriad of other cells.

As one cell changes it also changes its links with other cells. These link up with other cells which then also change and these link with other cells and so the process continues. Each time cells change they change the functional systems. I have already written about the concepts of Functional Systems in Chapter 14.

Obviously, the more cells which change and the more important the cells which change, the more likely the functional system is to change. It is like the ballot box in an election. The more votes which seek to change a system, the more likely it is

167

to bring about change. The factors which sway the millions of voters of different ages, personalities, economic backgrounds, social classes, philosophies etc., are extremely complex. The factors which bring about change in a functional system are probably equally complex.

Let me reiterate.

1   The changing of sensory functional systems can be through the senses of vision, hearing, touch, taste, smell, and from the sensors for balance and joint and muscle movement.

2   Changes in these sensory functional systems can alter the production of thought and memory.

3   Changes in thought alter the motor functional systems which bring about the millions of different movements of which our bodies are capable.

At the level of the brain cell even the most advanced neurological scientists are not able to give all the details of how our brains change. Fortunately we do not have to. In a way, much of what we see is a representation of our thoughts or someone else's thoughts.

The way we organise our environment is a reflection of the way we think, allowing for the fact that we are not free agents of change in our environment.

You arrange your home in the manner you want, taking into account the varying desires and strengths of all who live in the house. If you do not like the path to your door, or the position of the door, or the colour of the walls, or the wallpaper, you change your path or the position of your door or the colour to one which is to your liking.

If your brain is correctly organised to deal with the environment in which you live physically, mentally, socially and spiritually, you may be in a state of harmony,

If your brain is not organised for the environment or if the environment is changed too rapidly for your brain to adapt, it is likely that you will be under threat. You will be placed in a "fight or flight" situation with stress resulting, if you cannot resolve the problem. Your hot brain comes into action and dominates your thinking (see Chapter 5). Imagine if you are a city dweller, suddenly placed in a desert or a jungle. You would have few skills or functional systems relating to living in such an area and you would need to rapidly develop new skills or modify old ones to survive. You would be in a situation of cultural shock.

Dr. E. Le Winn, *Human Neurological Organisation* (Charles C. Thomas Springfield, Illinois, 1969) writes, "In large part the success or failure of the individual in relating to his environment depends on his neurological organisation." Le Winn defines neurological organisation as, "The process whereby the organism, subject to environmental forces, achieves the potential inherent in its genetic endowment."

In plain words, Le Winn considers that each person is in the process of becoming neurologically organised when the genetic gifts s/he possesses are brought to fruition within the imposed environmental limits.

In plainer words, it means that we are neurologically organised when the abilities we possess, flourish to the maximum in the environment.

This once again brings to our attention the age-old relationship between nature and nurture — between what is inherent in us and the changes in us that are wrought by the environment.

Leaving that question aside, there are several other very important matters which need attention. These are:

1 DOES THE NORMAL BRAIN REORGANISE IF THE ENVIRONMENT IS CHANGED?

This may seem a silly question. We all know that if we go to school our brains are changing. We all know that if we go to live in a foreign country and begin to learn the language our brain changes. Not only does our brain change in relation to language, it also changes with the other information placed into it. We learn where the new house is, where the transport routes are, where the closest and best shopping centre is situated, where the schools are, etc. We learn an enormous amount of relevant information. Our brain is now different from before. It is functioning in a different manner. To me this sounds reasonable and to most people it is reasonable. The academic scientific question is whether the brain changes STRUCTURE and FUNCTION. This change in your brain is dependent upon the concept of PLASTICITY.

Plasticity

Some people take a very broad view of plasticity which I personally hold as correct. Professor Richard Lerner, Professor of Child Development at Pennsylvania State University, in the preface of *On the Nature of Human Plasticity*, (Cambridge University Press,1984), writes of those who take a life span perspective of plasticity, "Those taking this perspective emphasize that the potential for change exists across life", and "They contend that change and the potential for change characterize life because of the plasticity of the processes involved in people's lives. From the level of biology to that of culture, these processes are presumed to be open to change — on the basis of both their inherent character and their reciprocal relations with other processes" and "The existence of plasticity is not a point of minor practical significance. If all levels of life are open to change, then there is great reason to be optimistic about the ability of intervention programmes to enhance human development."

One of the very important structures in the brain involved with plasticity is called the *Synapse*. It is the junction between two nerves where the message is transmitted from one nerve to the next. One way of imagining the synapse is to think of a corner where two or more roads meet. The roads can only be thought of as One Way Streets — just as the nerves can only carry message traffic in a one way direction. (This may, of course, be challenged in the future.)

Animal studies have shown that changing the environment can change the structure and function of the brain and the change is often in the number and the size and the enzyme activity of the synapse. Imagine road junctions which have to be enlarged, and possibly increased in number to handle more traffic.

Some of the pioneering work in animals was done on rats by Mark Rosenweig, Edward Bennett and Marian Diamond and was reported in *Scientific American* (Freeman, San Francisco, February 1972). These researchers asked the question,

169

"Does experience produce any observable change in the brain?", and they answered,

"Convincing evidence of such change has been found in the past decade. It has now been shown that placing an experimental animal in enriched or impoverished environment causes measurable changes in brain anatomy and chemistry." They also write, "Rats kept in a lively environment for 30 days show distinct changes in brain anatomy and chemistry compared with animals kept in a dull environment."

What they are saying is that the brain was changed by the effect of the environment.

They affirm their conclusions by the words, "Although the brain differences induced by the environment are not large, we are confident that they are genuine." This change in the brain is plasticity.

Commenting on the effect on the synapses they write, "Measurement of synaptic junctions revealed that rats from enriched environments had junctions that averaged approximately 50 per cent larger in cross section than similar junctions in littermates from impoverished conditions." (The latter however, had more synapses.)

D.Krech who worked with Rosenweig commented, "Although it would be scientifically unjustified to conclude at this stage, that our results do apply to people, it would, I think, be socially criminal to assume that they do not apply, and so assuming, fail to take account of the implications."

Dr Le Winn in *Human Neurological Organisation* equates the effects of increased function of the brain with what happens in other tissues. In other words, he considers that just as leg muscles enlarge if you undertake running every day, the brain increases in functional ability if you increase its workload up to an optimum. He writes," The principle that functioning of a tissue increases the size of its elements and the richness of its blood supply applies to the brain as much as to any other organ."

You might think that all this is academic. You could never be more wrong. There are still doctors, both neurologists and rehabilitationists who reject the whole concept of plasticity and will not even entertain the idea for discussion purposes.

If these doctors will not consider plasticity in the normal person, how do they think of plasticity as applied to the brain-injured person? They reject it out of hand. This then leads to the conventional thinking that;

NOTHING CAN BE DONE TO HELP THE PERSON WHO IS BRAIN-INJURED

If nothing can be done to help the brain-injured, they think, why waste time and resources on them? Let them be cast off, out of the health care system.

Fortunately this thinking is decreasing and recognised texts are now carrying the new message on plasticity. That is, that it may be possible to reorganise or rewire the brain by changing the environment.

2 DOES THE INJURED BRAIN REORGANISE IF THE ENVIRONMENT IS CHANGED?

This question is central to rehabilitation of the brain-injured. Those who assert that the brain of the brain-injured cannot change are denying that they have the function of plasticity. It is as if they consider that once a brain is injured it becomes rock hard and solid and is incapable of change. I do not know what scientific evidence there is for this view but I would hold the opinion that living tissue has the capacity to change.

Carl Cotman and James McGaugh from the University of California editing a book, *Behavioural Neuroscience* (Academic Press, New York,1980), write, "Studies on reactive synaptogenesis clearly demonstrate that the adult brain has an innate capacity to form new synapses in a highly selective manner." Reactive synaptogenesis means the reorganisation of the cell in response to a stimulus.

They also observe that "It is clear that the adult brain has the capacity to dynamically reorganise its circuitry, and after brain damage this plasticity must be taken into account."

Patients have demonstrated repeatedly that changing the environment can change their ability to function. Given the correct environment, changes occur in patients even years after the brain insult.

One young man, John, springs to mind immediately. With no movement in his left arm or left leg for two years, when placed on an intensive programme to restore function, he slowly regained the use of his left arm and is now slowly placing his hand on to his head. With his left leg, he is now capable of pushing a person or object away and has just started to walk in a walking frame.

This idea of change in the brain-injured is not foreign to many parents or to many doctors. Many people can tell stories of the change which came over someone brain-injured who, taken home and worked on with love and care by the family, has regained a significant amount of function.

One of my happiest memories relates to the "pedalling vegetable", a young man who was brain-injured and whose parents were told that he would be a vegetable. Recently I contacted the father of this person, and enquired how the young man was going. He informed me that his son was now riding an adult tricycle for 12 miles a day on the road. He finished off with the statement "Not bad for a vegetable!"

Sure enough, when I arrived at the home to check out the progress of this lad, having finished my medical examination, I asked for a demonstration of riding on the road. The patient was slowly led to the bike by his father walking in front of him with his arms outstretched. A crash helmet was fitted and with some help, Mark sat on the bike and slowly pedalled into the street, went for some distance and turned the bike around still sitting on it, and rode back. I was concerned about the brakes but soon found that not only could he brake, he could use the lever to change gear as well! Not bad for a vegetable.

While this regaining of function is likely to occur to a greater extent in the younger person, age is not an absolute barrier. Dr S.Finger comments in *Recovery from Brain Damage. Research and Theory* (Plenum Press, 1978), "There is evidence to suggest that a stimulating environment can also overcome some of the effects of brain lesions inflicted after sexual maturity."

Richard Lerner in his book on plasticity describes various researchers and writers who regard plasticity as "an ever present but declining phenomenon", and who write, "these data suggest that while the organism can be changed across life, it becomes increasingly more difficult to effect change: change requires a more intensive environmental stimulus, i.e., with age."

In other words, plasticity occurs to a greater degree in the young and reduces as a person becomes older.

Therefore, while canalization provides the direction that re-development will take, the extent of travel along the recovery pathway will be determined by the amount of irreversible damage as one factor, and the plasticity, or the ability to reorganise the brain as another.

3 THE IMPORTANCE OF THE EFFECTIVE STIMULUS IN THE PATIENT IN COMA

We already know a great deal about how to make a stimulus effective. If a young child is playing near the road, we may tell him/her to come away from the road. If this produces no response, we will raise our voice. If this produces no response we will move towards him/her and issue a threat. If this produces no response we will move to carry out the threat and take the child away from the roadside. This has already been discussed in Chapter 13 when I spoke about the episode in Wells in the U.K. I just wish to reinforce what I said there. Read through the list of Rules of Brain Function in that chapter again, for the procedure of making a stimulus effective is there.

4 THE CRITICAL TIME TO START WORK ON THE PATIENT WITH SEVERE BRAIN INJURY

We are all familiar with the concept of the critical time. We know that if we are to catch a plane, there is a certain time by which we must be at the airport. If we are late, unless the plane is delayed, we will miss it.

At school, dealing with the young, there appear to be critical times. These appear to be phases during which the child is sensitive to particular influences, whereas, at other stages of development, the child may be less sensitive, or even insensitive to the same influences.

J.P. Scott in *Early Experience and the Organisation of Behaviour*, (Belmont California Wadsworth, 1968), defines a critical time as "A time when a large effect can be produced by a smaller change in conditions than in any later or earlier period in life."

In the development of the young child, R.C. Sprinthall and N.A. Sprinthall (*Educational Psychology A Developmental Approach*, Third Edition, Addison-Wesley Publishing Company, 1981), make the statement about critical periods, "A great deal of research remains to be done in this important area. At this point there are few hard facts to indicate precisely when the various critical periods occur. We do know, however, that critical periods generally coincide with most rapid growth".

These words, applying to development in the young may equally well apply to the brain-injured. There is an extraordinary amount of research to be carried out to find the critical periods to intervene after brain trauma.

The time to commence the arousal of the patient in coma may be the first to be investigated. No one would suggest that this process should be undertaken when the patient is still in the life-threatened state, but it would seem reasonable that the sooner the patient can be aroused from coma and commenced on appropriate rehabilitation, the better may be the result.

So often in our present system, the approach has been to wait for the patient to wake up, hoping that this will occur. Most people do come out of coma spontaneously but this may be weeks, months even years after the accident and this time of non or minimal intervention may represent an opportunity to restore function which can never be fully regained.

This statement, of course, is difficult to prove or disprove but the fact that early intervention in an attempt to restore function in the stroke patient is now accepted and encouraged provides a parallel which should, at the very least, be explored.

The same situation occurs also with the baby who is brain-injured at birth, or the child who is developmentally disabled in some other way. The cry is now heard and is becoming stronger:

"Do not leave the child without an adequate attempt to restore function." This cry should also be heard in regard to the severely brain-injured, but the brain-injured are mute or can't speak adequately of their problems.

To observe a brain-injured person, with good intellectual abilities hampered by grossly impaired joints or muscle problems, frustratedly striving to regain movement of their joints and muscles, can only be viewed with anguish and compassion by the observer, along with horror that such a state should be allowed to occur within the framework of modern medicine or indeed within our civilization.

5   THE CRITICAL LEVEL OF INPUT

People frequently ask about THE programme for arousal from coma. They have some naive idea that there is one programme. When you check out the chapters in Section E, you will see that there are many programmes and many possible variations of each programme. It is like asking people what is food; there are so many foods each eaten in different proportions in the daily intake.

One thing which is extremely important, however, is that the input of stimuli, seeking to bring about changes in the brain, should be given at the right level. It is no good attempting to provide sophisticated stimuli to the injured brain when it is still incapable of processing the information. A parallel would be the giving of university mathematics to a toddler. There would be no point in it. It is important to stick to commonsense. If a patient is provided with an input which can be partly processed, but not fully, this may lead to confusion which if continued can only lead to frustration and to anger and to evidence of aggression. Ensure that for most of the input to a patient, the information is provided at a level which they can process.

SECTION E

THE THERAPY

It is the greatest
of all mistakes
to do nothing
because
you can only do
little.

Sydney Smith

CHAPTER 18

WHAT TO DO IN THE UNCONSCIOUS AND UNRESPONSIVE PATIENT

THE STAGE 1 PROGRAMME

Introduction

The following programmes are based on the pioneer work of Dr E. Le Winn from the Institute for the Achievement of Human Potential in Philadelphia, Sandlers and Brown (Consultants), of Philadelphia, Dr M. Dimancescu, Neurosurgeon of New York, Dr D. Clark, Director of the British Life Assurance Trust in the United Kingdom, and Mr Ian Hunter, Clinical Director of the Australian Centre for Brain-injured Children, Melbourne, Australia. None has consulted directly in the preparation of this book, however, and may not agree with all that follows.

If the patient is in coma and will not respond to anything you do to him or her, even using very painful measures, they are in the very deepest level of coma. On the Glasgow Coma Scale, they would be scored as 3. This is the very lowest score possible.

When the patient is in this condition, you have one aim: to get him or her out of unresponsive coma into a state of responsive coma. You may have to work very hard and consistently in an effort to achieve this goal.

The chances are that the patient will come out of coma for it is unusual for a person to stay at this low level of coma for a long period. In most instances, you will notice that the patient slowly starts to respond when things are done to them. The first responses are likely to be to pain. You may notice that they flinch when given an injection or when moved. You may notice some flickering of the eyelid or some deep breathing occurring at the time of the painful stimulus.

Usually, by the second week after a severe head injury, there is some obvious sign of a response. This may be only to pain. You will be pleased that this has occurred. But you will know from what has already been written, that it is important to receive information from the environment, using *all* our sense organs. It is not enough just to have the message coming to the patient's brain from the touch organs relaying pain, but he or she also needs messages to go to their brain from their eyes and their ears and from the nerves controlling their joints and muscles and also the nerves controlling balance.

So be happy when the patient does respond to pain, but remember that it is a very primitive response. By itself, it is not sufficient. No one can exist, and have any meaning in life, if they do not have the use of other senses and have a method of moving arms or legs or communicating to the world in some understandable manner. You will need to make sure that the patient recovers other ways of finding out about the environment through eyes, ears, other touch pathways of hot and cold, vibration, taste and smell.

You will need, therefore, to set up a programme for the patient to stimulate eyes, ears, skin, muscles, joints and balance mechanisms. The order of the programme will be arranged in *cycles*. It will need to be written down in a book in a way all can understand. You will need to provide the programme every day in the early stages and reduce it to six days per week in the later stages. You should always start off with a small amount and see the response of the patient. I would suggest half an hour each morning and afternoon for the first two days, and if all goes well, increase the amount by half an hour each day until you are providing about six hours per day after two weeks.

If you think that the programme is affecting the patient adversely, you should notify the ward sister who will contact the doctor if she is worried. You may have to stop for a day or two, or even longer, and then recommence. You will need to be guided by the attending doctor as to how long you should stop and when you should recommence.

If you feel the patient is coping but are asked to stop by the doctor, enquire about the reasons for this. I have usually found that the major reasons to hold the programme in abeyance relate to severe chest infections and difficulties over blood-pressure control, both of which can be serious and will need to be corrected before it is safe to continue the programme.

The following is a programme for the patient who is *not* responding. It provides input for vision, hearing, touch, pain, temperature, vibration, muscle and joint movement and balance mechanisms. Do not feel obliged to do every part of it. Do what can be done and forget the rest. It is likely that you are going to be involved in providing some care to the patient for months or even years, so always approach the programme from the point of view that if you cannot do one part initially or for a week or a month, there is still plenty to do. Those parts which you can't do now, can be done in the future.

Always remember that this programme must not in any way interfere with the normal medical and nursing and paramedical needs of the patient. Therefore, if you are in the middle of the programme and the doctor or nurse or physiotherapist or occupational therapist comes into the room, you should ask them if they wish you to stop. If they do, take note of where you were on the programme, cease what you are doing until they have finished their work, and then continue from where you left off. Do not antagonize the hospital staff by continuing the programme if they wish to examine the patient.

The *STAGE 1* programme will be set up in the following way:

THE PROGRAMME FOR VISION
THE PROGRAMME FOR HEARING
THE PROGRAMME FOR TOUCH
THE PROGRAMME FOR JOINT AND MUSCLE MOVEMENT
THE PROGRAMME FOR VESTIBULAR STIMULATION (BALANCE)

Each of these programmes will be split into
1. Aim
2. State of response
3. Stimulus used
4. Method of application
5. Timing of application
6. Duration and frequency of application
7. Contraindications (that is, things which you must be aware of which will not allow the programme to be given).

Go back to Chart 1 and copy from that chart onto this chart. This will be your reference chart.

CHART 1   SENSORY FUNCTION

	Visual	Auditory	Tactile
STAGE 1	No response	No response	No response
STAGE2	Pupillary response	Startle reflex	Extension flexion response
STAGE 3	Blink to touch, light, confrontation	Habituation	Withdrawal of limb
STAGE 4	Localize visual stimuli	Localizes auditory	Localizes tactile
STAGE 5	Eye contact Visual recognition	Comprehends auditory input	Discriminates tactile input

THE STAGE 1 PROGRAMME FOR VISION

Aim

The aim of the visual part of the programme in the unconscious and unresponsive patient is to attempt to bring about some constriction (making smaller) of the pupil by shining a light on to it.

177

State of Response

The size of the normal pupil varies depending upon the amount of light that it receives, as well as emotional and other factors. It usually varies from 2 mm up to about 8 mm. Normally, if the pupil is large, it will reduce in size (constrict) when a light is directed on it.

At this stage of coma you will see that the pupil is often larger than normal, and will either not constrict or will do so only very sluggishly. Sometimes you may need to use a magnifying glass to see if constriction occurs.

If the pupils are very small, this may be due to some of the drugs administered to help keep the intracranial pressure within normal limits. Sometimes the pupils are so small that they are called pinpoint pupils. An increase in intracranial pressure may also cause the pupils to become small. If you happen to notice this for the first time, especially if it is only in one eye, you should notify the ward sister immediately.

It is not unusual to have one pupil normal size and responding and the other enlarged and not responsive. In this case provide a programme for both pupils as though they were both non-responsive.

Stimulus Used

Usually when the doctor or nurse look at the pupils to see whether they are constricting or not, they use a penlight torch. This is a very small light source, and frequently you will find that the pupil will either not constrict or it will be difficult to see any movement. I, therefore, use a five-cell torch and can often get constriction with this, when I have failed to do so with a small penlight.

There have been occasions where this larger torch has failed to bring about any reaction, and I have used an electric spotlight of 100 watts, such as is used for outside lighting. Some people have expressed concern about the use of such a light. It is easy to test the effect of this light yourself. Close one eye and look for one second at a 100 watt light and you will soon see that it will not worry either you or the patient.

If the pupils are pinhole only, use the small torch.

Method of Application

Apply the light directly in front of the pupil by leaning over the bed or chair and putting the light in front of one eye at a time. Do not hold the light in front of the nose and attempt to stimulate both eyes together. The distance which you must hold the light from the eye is about 10-15 cm (4-6 in). If the room can be darkened, the contrast between the dark room and the light will be greater for the pupil. This darkening of the room is often of help.

Timing of Application

The light is held in front of the eye for one second, and then removed. It is best to do this by counting. Shine the light on to the eye and say *and one, and two, and three, and four.* Then swing the light back to the eye and do the same twelve times. Then move around the bed and do the same to the other eye. That is, you apply light to the eye for twelve times each minute. If only one eye is accessible to you, provide the stimulus to that eye.

Duration and Frequency of Application

The duration of application is one minute for each eye. The frequency is as required in the cycle.

Contraindications

Often patients with head injuries have some eye injury. If the eye has a patch or bandage over it, you must not disturb the dressing. If the eyelid is very swollen, as sometimes happens when blood and other tissue fluids drain down from the forehead, it is wise not to touch the eyelid, unless you have the ward sister's permission. An eyelid which will not open spontaneously is not a contraindication. Just hold the eyelid open with the finger and thumb of one hand and use the torch in the other hand. If you cannot open it, leave it shut and shine the torch towards the eye anyway.

THE STAGE 1 PROGRAMME FOR HEARING

Don't forget what has already been said about hearing. There appear to have been instances when the person considered to be in coma has been able to hear and comprehend some of the discussion at the bedside.

The potential for destructive comment under these circumstances, and the effect on the emotional state of the patient, may be very great. Every patient in coma should be considered to have the capacity to hear.

The following rules should be strictly adhered to:

1. Positive statements of encouragement only to be used in front of the patient.
2. All positive actions or reactions to be congratulated.
3. No negative or pessimistic statements to be made at the bedside.
4. All visitors to introduce themselves, or preferably be introduced by a person already familiar to the patient.
5. All people who are unfamiliar to the patient to state in clear terms why they are present and what they intend to do.
6. When any procedures are to be performed, the patient must be given information on who is performing the procedure, whether it will hurt and when, how long it will take, and what it is for.
7. All instructions and statements to be given in a clear, loud voice and in an unambiguous fashion.
8. No more than one person to be speaking at the one time.

Aim

The aim of stimulating the hearing mechanism of the patient is to obtain a response to noise. You want him or her to register, in some way, that a noise has been heard.

State of Response

When we hear a sudden loud noise, we jump or blink or grimace or start in some way. When the patient is in this low level of coma (that is, unconscious and unresponsive), he does not startle, blink or grimace at a sharp, loud noise. There is no response.

In most patients, however, if you look closely, you will see a response. It may be very small and, in the first instance, may just be that the patient will breathe more deeply or more rapidly. It seems to be unusual to lose all hearing ability; I have, however, seen unresponsive patients.

Stimulus Used

The stimuli used for hearing depend upon the giving of a single loud, clear sound for a short period of time. Loud horns, whistles, rattles, drums, blocks of wood are the easiest to obtain and also the most effective.

Klaxon-type horns, which have a rubber bulb at one end and can be squeezed firmly, are the best. When buying one, always try it out in the shop, since some of them are poorly made and fall to pieces, or fail to give a good penetrating sound. It is wise to buy two of them, so that you have a standby horn.

Whistles are easily obtained from a sports store. The ones we prefer are those used by referees in football or basketball games. They give a sharp, clear sound and are very dependable. There are also whistles with a variable pitch, which may be of value later. In the early stages it is best to stick to the referee whistle.

Rattles are more difficult to use. They are harder to control in an effort to give a sharp sound. The ones which have a rattle rotating on the end of a stick are probably the best, but make sure that you do not hit the patient when you swing.

Drums can give a measured beat and can be used quite successfully. You obviously need only a small child's drum and not one belonging to a regimental band.

Blocks of wood banged together will also make a definite sound. The blocks should be of hard wood, very smooth and about 15 cm long and 10 cm wide. If you fix a handle to the outside of them, it will save the fingers of the users.

Method of Application

You will use each of these different instruments one at a time and in rotation: in one cycle you will use the horn, in the next a drum, in the next a whistle, and so on.

The instrument is to be held about 30 cm away from the ear, and in the case of the horn in parallel with the side of the head. Do not point the horn directly at the ear, unless you obtain no response in any other way.

Timing of Application

The sound is made sharply and approximately every five seconds for one minute (that is, 12 times) on one side of the head, and then repeated on the other side of the head. The timing is not critical, so if you give the stimulus only 10 times per minute, do not be concerned.

Duration and Frequency

The duration and frequency is as required in the cycle.

Contraindications

Loud noises, quite rightly, are not welcomed in hospitals, especially where there are very sick patients in intensive care or in the high-dependency wards. You have to provide loud noise as part of the programme, so it is always wise to discuss it with the ward sister before you start. If you are in a single room, as many coma patients are, there is usually no great problem. You should show the ward sister what the extent of the noise is: it may not, in any way, intrude on the general running of the ward. If you are not able to work in a single room, or if the noise penetrates into the ward in any offensive manner, you may have to make a tape-recording of the sounds and use headphones on the patient.

If there are bandages or dressings around the head and ears, you must not disturb them in any way without the ward sister's permission. Often a bandage lightly covers the ear and can easily be lifted and placed above the ear. Do not be tempted to touch this until you have been given authority to do so.

THE STAGE 1 PROGRAMME FOR TOUCH

The capacity to feel touch is one our most primitive abilities. Our body surface is approximately two square metres, depending upon our size. Our skin is full of a remarkable number of nerve endings which can pick up any distortion or damage to the skin. Some parts of our bodies are particularly sensitive and we use them for feeling. Watch an infant and you will see how much information can be obtained when something is placed near the mouth. It is very likely that you can be given a small coin into the palm of your hand and be able to feel the difference between the two sides. You will be able to distinguish heads from tails, even with your eyes shut.

The soles of our feet are also well supplied with nerve endings. Some people who are unable to use their arms have trained their feet to be extremely receptive and able to feel almost as much as hands. The other areas of great sensitivity are in the armpit and the groin. We instinctively know that these areas need protection, and we have the touch sensitivity there to be able to detect any potential dangers.

The provision of pain to the patient is important. You might find this difficult to do. No one likes to give pain to another person. What you have to remember is that at this deep stage of coma, *the patient is not feeling the pain.* The next thing you must remember is that you need to wake the patient up. This is the important thing, and a small amount of pain is of little concern if this can be accomplished. You do not need to be cruel.

You must also remember that there are many times when pain is caused in medicine and in nature. Every person who has a surgical operation is likely to have a great deal more pain than you are likely to cause your patient. Yet few people refuse an operation because of the anticipated pain. Mothers giving birth to children often experience intense pain, but this incidence of pain does not seem to affect the birth rate. Many primitive races have initiation ceremonies which demand the provision of pain to the initiates.

Pain is not foreign to the human race. It is a part of it. If you are however, unable to use a painful stimulus, then you should be prepared to use the other stimuli and get someone else to provide the painful ones.

Aim

The aim of the touch part of the programme is to provide a stimulus to the unconscious and unresponsive patient by the use of touch, in order to bring about some movement.

State of Response

In this state of unresponsive coma the patient does not react.

You will already have seen the emphasis that has been placed on the importance of the patient responding to pain. While pain is the most usual stimulus to bring about a response, the patient may not respond to pain, but may respond to a vibrator or to ice.

Stimulus Used

Pain on skin

Painful pressure can be applied either by pinching the skin on a part of the body or limbs, using the finger and thumb, or by squeezing a part of the body between the thumb and the back of a nailbrush.

The input of pain is decreased as the patient becomes increasingly aware, to the point of cessation if it is causing hurt to the patient.

Pain with hair-pulling

Relatives will often do this to the hair on the head or beard, but not to other parts of the body. If you try pulling the hair on your arms, you will see that it is not too painful. I think that antagonism to hair-pulling is developed in us when we are children, and are told that it is wrong to pull hair.

Pain with pressure on muscle

This is very effective, especially on the thick muscle bodies of the limbs. You can either grip the muscle body between your fingers and thumbs, or use a nailbrush and squeeze the muscle between the nailbrush and your thumb.

182

Touch

Touch can be either light or heavy. Light touch is most unlikely to produce any response with the patient in deep coma, so do not bother with it at this stage. Heavy touch is putting your hands heavily on, and applying pressure to, different parts of the body.

Another excellent method is to use a hard nailbrush and scratch the body and limbs with this. If you use this, be prepared for some marks on the skin surface and be especially careful around the face in the young or women. If the skin is fragile and likely to be damaged, do not use this method. I recall a 16-year-old patient who was inadvertently scratched on the face to the degree of actually drawing blood. It was very difficult explaining to his mother and aunts why this had occurred. When you do use a brush, always have some skin cream to apply to any scratched areas.

Temperature changes

The body surface is very susceptible to temperature changes in our environment. We normally balance heat loss or gain by the use of our clothing, discarding it when we become hot and replacing it when we become cold. The mass of temperature receptors in our skin, as well as the temperature of our blood, lets our brain know when we should modify our clothing so we can control our temperature exchange with our environment. We can also discern, when we are conscious, the area in which heat loss or gain has occurred and also the size of the area involved. If we have cold feet, we soon take action to put on thicker socks or ug boots etc.

Ice is the stimulus which should be used. Obviously you will not provide total body exposure to the ice, since you do not want the patient to get cold. Use it, therefore, in small areas at a time. It is easily obtainable in most hospitals as cubes, and these can be placed in a small plastic bag about the size of a hand. Another method is to make ice-blocks on a stick. Heat is generally not used because of the obvious dangers of burning or scalding. Some people do apply warm sponges to parts of the body, especially to joints if they are painful. This appears to work well, but make sure that there is not too much water in the sponge and check the temperature on yourself first.

Vibration

Vibrators can be bought from a pharmacy. Often the ones first offered are not sufficiently strong and tend to fall to bits over a week or so of intensive use. Commercial vibrators, such as those used in beauty salons, are best. You may need to get your pharmacist or drug store to make a special order for one. Also ensure that the cord will be long enough. For safety reasons, many hospitals do not like extension leads.

Method of Application

All of the suggested stimuli are used by direct application to the body surface, especially the face, the lips, around the mouth, ears, head, hands, fingers, chest,

183

abdomen, groin and all sensitive areas. Often the back is inaccessible for much of the time, but it can be used when the patient is in the shower or being sponged in bed.

You do not need to provide constant pain or tug at the hair for a long time. Just pull the hair and let go. The same applies when you are providing the painful stimulus: give it for a second or so, and then move to another part of the body.

When you use the vibrator or ice or nailbrush, go over the face on both sides first. Then commence a continuous sweep from the neck down over the right shoulder and over the front of the right arm and wrist and hand, and continue along the back of the right hand, wrist and arm and across the neck and on to the front of the left arm down to the hand and back in the same way as for the right arm. Next move on to the chest and go from one side to the other till it has all been covered. Then go on to the abdomen (stomach) and move across it, until it has been covered.

Next move on to the right groin and down the front of the leg to ankle and the toes, and then up the back of the leg to the buttock. Then go on to the left leg and down to the foot in the same manner. It is unlikely that the first few times of doing this you will be able to finish the total available body surface in five minutes. Do not be concerned. With practice you will soon be able to achieve it.

Every time you move on to a new part of the body or move down a limb, you tell the patient in a loud, clear voice where you are. You call him or her by name and say, "I am moving the ice down the right side of your face and am now going on to the left side of your face. I am now moving the ice on to your right shoulder", and continue for the whole body.

Some physiotherapists may be concerned that these stimuli should not be applied to certain surfaces of the arms and the legs. This opinion should not necessarily prohibit the provision of these stimuli in the early stages, until the patient is out of coma. The matter needs further consideration and review.

Duration and Frequency of Application

You should provide the stimulus for five minutes at any one time. It is important to change the stimulus in each cycle. The frequency will be as required by the cycle.

Contraindications

If there are any dressings on any part of the body, you must not disturb them in any way without the ward sister's permission. The same applies where the patient has a fracture and has a limb in a splint. Do not disturb without permission. If the patient has a limb in plaster, it is usually acceptable to touch those areas of the limb above and below the plaster, but it is always wise to check with the sister first.

THE STAGE 1 PROGRAMME FOR JOINT AND MUSCLE MOVEMENT

Our brain has a massive amount of stimuli presented to it from our joints and muscles, as well as our skin. Our brain needs to know precisely where each of our joints is at any given moment, so that the position of our body can be controlled in regard to the environment. If we need to fight or flee for our survival, we must have joint and muscle control constantly ready to take survival actions. The nerve pathway carrying these inputs from the muscle and joints to the brain is called the *proprioceptive* pathway. This proprioceptive input to our brain is one of the most primitive sensory inputs, along with touch and our balance mechanisms (vestibular inputs).

Aim

The aims of providing joint and muscle movement are;

1. To attempt to awaken the brain in the unconscious and unresponsive patient
2. To stimulate the part of the brain which receives nerve impulses from the joints and muscles and
3. To attempt to prevent the joints and muscles from becoming abnormally tight.

Stimulus Used

Movement of all accessible joints by someone is of paramount importance. This is best done under the tuition and supervision of the hospital's Physiotherapy Department. The standard routine is for the physiotherapists to instruct the relatives in the provision of this stimulus. If there is no physiotherapist available, you should ask the ward sister either to show you or delegate someone to show you. Do not move joints and limbs without guidance unless there is no one to show you.

Method of Application

The movements should be performed in reference to a joint chart, so that all accessible joints are moved. This includes the neck, the arms, the wrists, the fingers, the hips, the knees, the ankles and the toes. The hospital should be able to provide a joint chart.

Duration and Frequency of Application

The range of movements should be given for ten minutes at any one time in the cycle.

This range of movement is maintained during the whole of the coma-arousal programme, until spontaneous movement becomes established. Even then it may be continued for months after the patient is out of coma.

Contraindications

Obviously those limbs which have dressings on them, or which may be fractured, should not be moved or can only be moved with the permission of the ward sister.

On no account should you force a limb into a movement. If the limb is stiff, you must first check with the physiotherapist or ward sister and seek their advice.

Many people express a worry that it is unwise to move the head of the patient, since there may be the possibility of neck damage. It is always wise to check with the ward sister or doctor or physiotherapist before moving the head. The relatives and friends do not usually commence this work until the patient is out of the life-threatened state, by which time a period of 10 to 14 days has already elapsed. During this time the patient would have had a neck X-ray and would have had the head moved many times by medical and nursing staff. It is still wise to check each day before any movement is attempted.

Sometimes physiotherapists like to use what are known as inhibition plasters. These are plasters of Paris which are placed on an arm or leg to try and prevent contractures of the limbs. It is hoped that by their use the joints can be kept in a more normal position. Unless they can be shown to be of use, they may be a serious disadvantage. They can certainly prevent the patient receiving good body movement and balance and touch stimulation.

In my experience these plasters are a disadvantage and are often a cause of conflict between those physiotherapists who advocate their use and those people who oppose their use.

The decision finally must be made by the next of kin. Are they after a functioning limb or a functioning brain? If they had to choose between the two, which would they take? Most people would prefer a functioning brain, if this can be achieved and would gladly dispense with inhibition plasters. In other words, it is better to do everything to get the patient awake using all the limb movement which can be obtained rather than leaving a limb encased in plaster and being unable to use it to send the proprioceptive messages to the brain.

THE STAGE 1 PROGRAMME FOR VESTIBULAR STIMULATION

The word vestibular relates to balance. It is a very primitive and important sense. The vestibular programme is often hard to administer to patients in coma, because people are worried about moving the patient too much. It should be provided only when the doctor says it is safe to move the patient.

Most hospitals realize the importance of putting the brain-injured patient into a sitting position in a chair. Some have not, however, learnt of the value of this approach and will keep the patient lying in bed for weeks or months without any real movement stimulation. Some of the drugs which are used can also immobilize the patient. In my opinion, also, the use of bean-bags for children with brain injury should be discouraged.

Much of the following is dealt with in more detail in Chapter 22, What to do in the Unconscious/Conscious and Responsive Patient — Motor Output.

Aim

To provide the unconscious and unresponsive patient with an input to the balance mechanisms of the brain in an attempt to awaken the patient and to stimulate those parts of the brain concerned with balance.

Stimulus Used

The person should be upright, so that the head can be held up. This requires help to support the head.

Method of Application

The patient should be in the upright position, sitting in a chair, as much as possible. The lying-down position is one of sleep, not arousal. Much of the visual and hearing and touch part of the programme can be carried out while the patient is sitting in a chair.

Head movements should be performed. These movements should include up and down movements, movement to the side and turning movement. None of these movements is to be forced. Just do them gently, without pushing or exerting too much pressure. If there is any concern about these movements, the ward sister should be notified.

At other times the patient should be placed on the edge of the bed in an upright position with the feet overhanging. This manoeuvre often needs three people, one on each side of the patient and one kneeling on the bed at the back, supporting the patient and stopping him or her from falling backward. The patient can then be turned from side to side and rotated around a vertical axis.

The tilt-table should be used for short periods of time as soon as the patient can safely cope with it.

When it is reasonable to do so, the patient should be placed on a mat on the floor where rolling and rocking of the whole body should be provided. If this cannot be done, it is often possible, if the condition of the patient allows it, to rock and roll on the bed.

Duration and Frequency of Application

Sitting in a chair should be increased from half an hour on the first day to up to six hours per day. Head movements should be for five minutes every cycle. Sitting on the edge of the bed should be provided at least for five minutes three times daily. The tilt-table should commence at five minutes' duration at a small angle to the horizontal and work slowly up to full elevation. Rocking and rolling should be carried out, if possible three times per day.

Contraindications

If the patient has trouble with blood pressure, it is wise not to move him or her without permission. Also, a limb with a fracture, especially if it is in a sling, can make any movement difficult.

DO NOT GET THE PATIENT OUT OF BED WITHOUT THE WARD SISTER'S PERMISSION.

It is also important for you to remember that the initial movements related to balance and gravity can be very discomforting to the patient, who has no control over his or her own body movement. It is of great importance, therefore, that when any awareness has developed, none of these manoeuvres should be performed without the presence of a relative who has the ability to calm and reassure the patient.

THE PROGRAMME FOR TASTE AND SMELL

It is always dangerous to attempt to give taste or smell stimuli at this stage. The patient has either a tube through the nose into the windpipe or a tracheostomy tube in place. In either event the mouth is a dangerous place in an unconscious patient for untrained people to be fiddling with. It is better to leave these two stimuli until a later time when the patient is more responsive.

SETTING UP THE PROGRAMME FOR THE UNCONSCIOUS AND UNRESPONSIVE PATIENT — THE STAGE 1 PATIENT

You will use the following programme for vision, hearing, and touch until there is evidence that the patient has a response to that stimulus which becomes constant.

This means that if the pupil starts to constrict to a 5-cell torch, you can go on to Stage 2 of the visual programme. If the patient responds to the hearing stimulus by giving a start, you can go on to the Stage 2 of the hearing programme. If the patient withdraws the limbs to a touch stimulus, you can place him or her on to a Stage 2 programme for touch.

The range of movement and vestibular stimulation will be used through most stages of the programme.

THE CYCLE FOR STAGE 1

STIMULUS USED	EQUIPMENT	TIME
Vision	5-cell torch or 100W light	2 min.
Hearing	Horn or rattle or whistle or drum or wood blocks	2 min.
Touch	Pressure, hair-pulling, heavy touch, nailbrush, or ice or vibrator	2 min.
Proprioception	Range of movement	10 min.
Vestibular	Rock and roll on bed or sit up on edge of bed	10 min.

If you allow say 30 minutes to do each cycle, allowing for change in position, you can do two cycles each hour. Start off with a cycle in the morning and the afternoon, and if all goes well, increase by another cycle in the morning and the afternoon until you are reaching 6 hours or 12 cycles per day.

Set the programme up on a chart on the wall beside the bed, and tick off each time you complete the activity listed. Do not be discouraged if you do not get any responses for days or even weeks. When you do get a response, write it in the diary. Keep all the records of the programme, so that you can refer back to them.

Vary the programme with regard to hearing and touch in the following manner, working cycle 1 followed by cycle 2 followed by cycle 3 etc.

	Vision	Hearing	Touch	Range of Movement	Vestibular
1.	Light	Horn	Pressure	Full range	Head movement
2.	Light	Rattle	Hair pull	Full range	Roll
3.	Light	Whistle	Heavy touch	Full range	Rock
4.	Light	Drum	Nailbrush	Full range	Sit on bed
5.	Light	Blocks	Ice/Vibrator	Full range	Head movement

Then commence the cycles again.

CHAPTER 19

WHAT TO DO IN THE UNCONSCIOUS AND

RESPONSIVE PATIENT — VISION

The therapy is changed when the patient responds. Because there may be a different level of response for sight, hearing and touch, each of these will be dealt with separately, using the same basic approach in Chapter 18.

STAGES 2, 3, 4, 5

When you feel that there is a response when light is shone into the eye of the patient, the patient is not in the unresponsive state. This means that progress has been made, and it is time to alter the stimuli being given.

Before you read this chapter, you must read Chapter 18, taking note especially of the sections marked CONTRAINDICATIONS. The contraindications will often apply to patients who are responsive, but still in coma. You must not disregard them. If you have any doubts, you should seek the advice of the ward sister. Always go back and study Chapter 18 when you are dealing with the patient who is in any stage from Stage 2 to Stage 4.

Do not forget, I have stressed constantly, that patients coming out of coma can vary tremendously from day to day, and from the morning to the afternoon. They also vary a great deal depending on who is with them, what drugs or other treatment they are receiving, and whether they are constipated or not. Sometimes they are just tired, and this can affect their performance and responses markedly.

As a result it is quite possible that a patient may be doing the things listed in Stage 4 in the morning but may only be doing Stage 2 things in the afternoon: or may be doing well one day and poorly the next. There is no sudden change from stage to stage as the patient improves. It is a gradual change which is often measured only in weeks, not in days. This is no different from a child gaining a skill, such as riding a bike. The first few times they may fall off, but as they continue, performance improves and the number of falls decreases. It is the same for us as we learn a skill, whether it is typing or bricklaying: we become better with practice. But we also vary from day to day in how well we do things, depending on whether we are tired, whether we are surrounded by people we like, etc. The brain-injured do the same. It is just that they cannot tell us why they are performing well one day and not the next. We have to be tolerant and patient and help to work this out with them.

If you have filled in the questionnaire in Chapter 9, and have identified the stage that the patient is in, it is time for you to work out their programme. This working-out of the programme is not critical. In other words, no one can be absolutely sure what is happening in the brain of the patient. What you have to do is be reasonable. You must identify as closely as you can the right STAGE from the questionnaire, and then mark in this chapter the correct STAGE of the therapy for vision, and write the activities up into a programme of action.

Again your programme of action is not critical. If you gave three minutes to vision instead of two minutes, it would not make any difference. If you held the light at 8 cm instead of 10 cm, it would not make any difference. Do not be worried about minor things in this programme. What is given is a guide, which can be varied depending upon the patient, his responses and the giver of the therapy.

THE PROGRAMME FOR VISION

The recovery of visual abilities is developed along a series of milestones which have been dealt with in Chapter 2, Measuring the Patient's Condition and What it Means, and Chapter 11, The Growth of Awareness and Return of Sensation. They are identified here for ease of reference while you select the appropriate programme.

STAGE 1	NO REACTION OF PUPIL TO LIGHT
STAGE 2	SOME PUPILLARY REACTION TO LIGHT
STAGE 3	BLINK REFLEX TO TOUCH, LIGHT, OBJECT.
STAGE 4	SOME CONTROLLED EYE MOVEMENT. LOCALIZING, FOLLOWING AND FIXATING ON LIGHT AND/OR OBJECT
STAGE 5	EYE CONTACT. DISCRIMINATION, INITIALLY COARSE PROGRESSING TO FINE.

You should read right through this chapter before you commence visual work. While I have split it up into the different stages, this should not stop you experimenting with each programme. In other words, if you want to try Stage 5 methods in Stage 3 or Stage 4, you should do so.

STAGE 1

This stage has been dealt with in the previous chapter on the unconscious and unresponsive patient.

STAGE 2

Aim

The aim is:

To get the eyelids to blink when a bright light or an object is directed towards the eye.

191

State of Response

The pupil will constrict, usually to a penlight torch, but will not move towards the stimulus. The eyelids will not blink when a bright light is shone on the eye.

Stimulus Used

The usual stimulus is a torch. TV can also be used.

Method of Application

Shine the light directly across the front of the pupil in a vertical, horizontal and diagonal plane, at a distance of 10-15 cm. Some people refer to this as an * (asterisk pattern). Another way is to think of the spokes of a wheel and follow those in your imagination, always coming back to the centre point or axle before you move in any direction.

In the case of TV, make sure that the TV is directed towards the patient and at a normal distance, and ensure that the volume is a little above what is normally used. The use of TV at this early stage may be seen as premature, but it should at least be tried.

Timing of Application

Five seconds to each eye with a five-second interval between each application, that is, application of light to the eye at the rate of six times per minute.

Do not leave the TV on all the time.

Duration and Frequency of Application

The duration of the stimulation is one minute for each eye. The frequency is as required in the cycle.

STAGE 3

Aim

To move the visual abilities of the patient into Stage 4, so that the eyes and forehead will fix on a light or an object.

State of Response

The pupil will constrict to a torch. The eyelids will blink to a touch, light and object.

Stimulus Used

The usual stimulus provided is coloured light of different types. This may be flashing and have a noise associated with it: for example, a ray gun. There is a whole range of children's toys which combine flashing lights and sound. Many of these should be obtained and used, varying the toy, but seeking constantly the one which produces the most results.

The other important stimulus is television. Do not leave the TV on all day, but select programmes which the patient has previously known and liked, and show those.

Method of Application

Lights should be placed directly across the face of the patient in a vertical, horizontal and diagonal plane from outside the body perimeter. This should be at a distance of 15-20 cm. The distance may be varied to several metres away from the patient. Always move the light slowly, talking as you move it to tell the patient where it is.

Position the TV so that the patient must make an effort to look towards the screen. Do not place it in an impossible position, though, and if the patient is obviously tired and wishes to watch a favourite programme, put the TV in the easiest place for them.

Duration and Frequency of Application

The duration of applying lights to the eyes is two minutes, and for watching TV thirty minutes in the early evening.

Frequency of application is as required in the cycle.

STAGE 4

Aim

To move the patient's visual abilities into Stage 5, where the patient is making eye contact, appearing to recognise faces or photographs or words.

State of Response

The pupil will constrict. The eyes or head may turn towards a stimulus and will localize and will fix the gaze on it for a short period of time. While this period of time will be fleeting initially it will increase in duration as the response becomes more established. In many patients the ability to move the eyes becomes apparent but they are often, because of weakness or increased muscle tension, unable to move their head to either side. Do not forget also that many patients are unable to move an eye to one side or towards the middle, because the nerve to the eye muscle has been damaged.

Stimulus Used

Photographs

The photographs that you show to the patient should be large, well coloured, distinct, preferably with much identifiable red and yellow in large amounts. People

193

should be shown as individuals or in small groups: that is, no more than three people per photograph. Especially use photographs of people, places and animals which are familiar to the patient. It is good to use photographs which have a strong emotional involvement.

Words

Do the same as for photographs. Use the name of the patient and the names of close family, mother, father, brothers, sisters, aunts and uncles, grandparents, friends, pets, places, sporting personalities, politicians, teachers. When you make up these words, use letters which are at least three centimetres high. Use a red colour on a yellow piece of cardboard. Make the letters thick, so they stand out well.

Television

TV can be used for longer periods up to one to two hours in the evening, selecting those shows to which the patient really reacts well. Do not overdo it, however, and do not substitute it for the other work periods.

Faces

We use our eyes constantly when we look at people. While at a distance we may only see their shape or outline, as we get closer to them we start to seek out their face. We then always direct our eyes towards their eyes. We make eye contact. This is the what we do normally every day. Eye contact is of great importance.

In my experience, when eye contact commences, it often appears the patient is saying that the "channel of communication is open", and that they are now conscious. At first, eye contact may be only fleeting. It may just be there for a second, but it is very important.

Method of Application

Photographs, words, faces should be placed in front of the patient in the early stages. Words and photographs should be in groupings of ten. When seeking eye contact, the face and eyes of the observer must attempt to engage the eyes of the patient. At the same time the patient is also told to look at the eyes of the observer.

Do not hold the objects too far away or too close. About half an arm's length from the eyes of the patient is good. Always show the photographs and words in a good light. Make sure that the blinds of the room are open and have the light shining as much as possible on to the photograph or word. If the patient normally wears spectacles, use them.

Varying the position of the TV in the room is worth doing as it forces the patient to change the angle of vision and may encourage them to use their eye muscles better.

In the early stages, while the patient is coming out of coma, they will not make eye contact. You may place your face in front of theirs, and you will get the feeling that they are looking "through" you, that they are not focusing on you. You will feel that their gaze is passing right into you without making any connection with your eyes. Place your face in front of theirs and attempt to hold their gaze. Do not be put off because you cannot initially gain the gaze from them. Persevere!

Duration and Frequency of Application

Use the photographs and words for two minutes. Do not hold them in front of the patient for more than a few seconds each. The photographs and words should be used very much as you would use flashcards with children. Eye contact should also be sought for a period of two minutes. The frequency of application is as required in the cycle.

STAGE 5

When the patient can localize a stimulus, fix on to it, pursue it and make eye contact, it may be assumed that he or she is out of coma. It is important constantly to increase the range and variety of photographs, cards, and words, so that the patient will relearn to discriminate visually. You must make it interesting. If patients start to turn away from what you are offering them, you may be boring them. You should find more interesting objects, pictures, etc., at which they can look. Professional help of some type would be advantageous. It may be worth seeking an opinion from a schoolteacher with an interest in special education.

CHAPTER 20

WHAT TO DO IN THE UNCONSCIOUS AND

RESPONSIVE PATIENT — AUDITORY

From the questionnaire in Chapter 9, you must mark to which stage the patient has progressed. You must then find the correct level in this chapter for hearing.

Read through this whole chapter and then mark in the correct therapy for the patient on your Programme Sheet.

As with vision, do not be afraid to try Stage 4 material at an earlier stage. It will not harm the patient.

Recovery of hearing appears to go through a set pattern as function improves. These milestones have been dealt with in a previous chapter.

The Levels of Hearing

STAGE 1	NO REACTION
STAGE 2	STARTLE, BLINK OR GRIMACE PRESENT SOME UNDERSTANDING OF TONE, ETC.
STAGE 3	WITHDRAWAL OF HEAD AWAY FROM NOISE, HABITUATION
STAGE 4	LOCALIZES SOUNDS, SOME INDICATION OF AUDITORY AWARENESS
STAGE 5	SOME COMPREHENSION OF SPEECH

STAGE 1

This stage has been dealt with in the patient who is unconscious and unresponsive in Chapter 18. Please refer to that section.

STAGE 2

Aim

To move the hearing abilities into Stage 3, the reflex survival stage, where withdrawal of the head or eyes away from a threatening stimulus, and habituation occur.

196

State of Response

The patient will startle, grimace or blink. When this occurs, it is assumed that there are some mechanics of hearing present and that the initial reflex stage has been reached.

Stimulus Used

1. As in the previous stage a loud horn, whistle, rattle, drum, blocks of wood, etc., are used.
2. Taped *environmental sounds*. Person whose voice is familiar to the patient. In one patient, a soldier, the voice of his RSM bellowing orders was used to good effect. Schoolchildren may benefit from tapes of their classmates. Noises of animals — dogs, cows, horses, etc. — transport noises of planes, cars, trucks, trains and work noises of phones, machines, etc. are all worth trying.
3. *Taped music*. While taped music may not be as good as a live production of sound, it may still be useful. The music should be appropriate to the patient's age and musical tastes. We have found that Vivaldi is not often appreciated by the young, and conversely that the older person is not enamoured with some modern music. In some patients the playing of specific musical notes while each is identified may be of benefit.

The use of music needs to be explored more fully. Professor Manfred Clyne of Sydney Conservatorium of Music has described the importance of music in our emotional lives in his book, *Sentics: The Touch of the Emotions* (Doubleday, 1977). Much of his knowledge would be applicable to these comatose and responsive patients.

4. *Speech*. In every section of the programme it is important to talk to the patient. This is best done by a variety of people, and it has been stressed that during the programme the patient should be told what is happening to him or her and also what to do. There should be one person, preferably a close relative or friend, who comes each day to let the patient know what is happening in the world that he knew, what his friends are doing, what is happening in sport, music, politics and anything else which is of interest to the patient. This may only take up a matter of minutes in the first instance, but will increase in length as the patient responds. Often people are not sure what they should say. It is usually best to make a list of topics for talking and take it as a script for guidance.

Method of Application

1. Position horn at the side of the head, directed away from the ear, and at a distance of 30 cm.

2 and 3. Via the tape-deck and earphones.

4. Follow the guidelines on speech given in Chapter 11.

Timing of Application

1. 12 times per minute.
2. Environmental sounds may be played at set times during the day.
3. Rhythmic music can be used as a routine during the range of motion exercises. There may also be a set type of music provided prior to sleep.
4. Usually about mid morning for 10-15 minutes.

Duration and Frequency of Application

Basic sounds one minute to each ear. Music as per above. Speech as above. Frequency of application is as per the cycle.

STAGE 3

Aim

To help the patient move into Stage 4, where he will localize sounds by turning his eyes or head towards the sound.

State of Response

The patient will withdraw the head away from a threatening sound. He or she will also habituate to the sound if it continues. If the horn is blown repeatedly and the startle reflex disappears, the patient is habituating. The patient may also begin to show signs of pleasure or discomfort when the environmental or music tapes are played. It is often difficult to pick up this stage, as the patient may be unable to turn the head away from noise which is irritating.

Stimulus Used

The use of loud noises, such as horns and drums and whistles near the patient, is discontinued, since it may become counter-productive. Loud noises produced at a distance from the patient will still be needed. The tape-recording of the voices of familiar people, environmental noises and music are continued as in the previous stage.

Method of Application

Loud noises at a distance from the patient, however, are important to try to get the patient to turn the head or eyes towards the noise. Attempts by the relatives to call the patient and seek a response from different sides of the bed and at a distance are encouraged, to see if the patient is localizing sound. Children familiar to the patient are often very good at getting a response where no one else can. It may be that their voices are more penetrating and shrill, or that they are just more noisy and not worried about being quiet in a hospital.

The tape decks are used as before.

STAGE 4

Aim

To move the patient into Stage 5, the stage of auditory discrimination, with some understanding of speech and, if possible, obeying a command.

State of Response

The patient will localize a sound. Eyes and/or head will turn towards the sound. The patient may discriminate between the tones of voice and react differently to different voices.

Stimulus Used

The full range of stimuli continues to be used with an emphasis on those people and stimuli which get the best results.

Method, Duration and Frequency of Application

As before.

STAGE 5

It is very likely that the patient is, in some way, obeying a simple command, such as to move an arm or leg or squeeze a hand. (Always be careful about the interpretation of this action: it may be a grasp reflex.)

Increasing ability to discern and understand may be gained by constantly varying the hearing stimuli in an interesting way to the patient. Additional help which can be given in the comprehension of voice and music, etc., is a matter of continuing education. Once again the services of a professional may be sought.

All the methods of speech, music, tapes, etc., which can be used should be made available to the patient.

CHAPTER 21

WHAT TO DO IN THE UNCONSCIOUS AND RESPONSIVE PATIENT — TOUCH

Before you read this chapter, return to Chapter 18 and go through it carefully with a marking pen. Most of what is contained there relates to the patient in all the stages as s/he comes out of coma.

The stages with touch stimuli may be briefly identified as:

STAGE 1	NO REACTION
STAGE 2	EXTENSION / FLEXION PATTERN
STAGE 3	LOCAL WITHDRAWAL OF LIMB
STAGE 4	LOCALIZATION
STAGE 5	DISCRIMINATION OF STIMULUS

Much of the information about these stages has already been presented in Chapter 2, Measuring the Patient's Condition and What it Means, and in Chapter 11, The Return of Sensation. It would be wise for you to read the relevant parts of those chapters again.

Do not forget that the following factors, which compromise body movement, unless absolutely necessary, are seen as counter productive:

1. Intensive drug therapy; which places the patient back into an obliterated state.
2. Inhibitory plasters; which prevent spontaneous movement and block nerve impulses from the skin, muscles and joints.
3. Body restrainers.
4. Traction apparatus.

STAGE 1

The programme for Stage 1, for the patient who is unconscious and unresponsive, has already been dealt with in Chapter 18.

Stimulus Used

The stimuli used in all stages are pain, hair-tugging, pressure on muscles, ice, vibrator.

Method of Application

Direct application is to the total body surface; the face, especially the lips, around the eyes, ears, head, hands, fingers, abdomen, groin and all sensitive bony areas (see Chapter 18).

It is important for the providers of the programme to announce what stimulus is being used, and on what portion of the body, in a loud clear voice: for example, I am applying ice to the back of your hand.

STAGE 2

Aim

To see if the patient can be moved from the generalized type response into Stage 3, the withdrawal stage.

State of Response

There is flexion or extension of the limb or limbs.

Stimulus Used

The stimuli used are pain, hair-tugging, pressure on muscles, ice, vibrator. These are alternately used in each cycle.

Method of Application

Direct application to the total body surface, the face especially the lips, periorbital regions, ears, head, hands, fingers, abdomen, groin and all sensitive bony areas (see Chapter 18).

Duration and Frequency of Application

Duration of application is ten minutes. The frequency is as required in the cycle.

Contraindications

If the extension/flexion is strong and generalized, it is frequently wise to withdraw for a period of days and then retest. It is also wise to

1. Check whether the patient is feverish.
2. See if the patient is constipated. It is not unusual for a constipated patient to spasm.
3. Ask the relative who has the best rapport with the patient to provide a modified form of the stimulus to the patient, for a brief period providing constant reassurance. It is best for this to be done when the patient has had a good night and is fresh in the morning.

STAGE 3

Aim

To take the patient from the local withdrawal stage to Stage 4, the Stage of Localization.

State of Response

The patient will withdraw the arm or leg to which the stimulus is applied.

Stimulus Used

Painful stimuli are ceased. The ice may be reduced in intensity and extent. Hand brushing and massage are appropriate stimuli in this stage.

Method of Application

As above.

Duration and Frequency of Application

The duration of the application is ten minutes. The frequency is as required in the cycle.

STAGE 4

It should be noted that spontaneous/ritualistic movement often becomes apparent between Stage 3 and Stage 4. It is suggested that at this time the patient has a developing awareness of his or her predicament. It is also suggested that the patient may be indicating by body language that he or she does not like what is occurring, and that the intrinsic drive within them is forcing them to seek change. They may, therefore, be labelled as aggressive.

Aim

To move the patient into Stage 5, where the patient can identify where and what the stimulus is. It is often also at this stage that voluntary control of a muscle group becomes obvious. This really means that when the patient is asked to perform a movement, he or she will obey. Do not forget about the "lag" time which frequently occurs in these patients.

State of Response

There is localization of the stimulus. The head or eyes may be turned towards the stimulus. The hand may reach out and push the stimulus away.

Stimulus Used

The vibrator and ice may be maintained, but reduced. Massage, etc., is used.

Method of Application

As above.

202

Duration and Frequency of Application

The duration of application is ten minutes. The frequency is as required in the cycle.

STAGE 5

The patient can indicate what the stimulus is and where it is. It is important that a body map of response to stimuli should be made, so that areas of deficiencies may be identified and an attempt made to correct them. The deficiencies may be for ice, or touch, or vibrator, etc.

Programme for Proprioception

Passive movement of all accessible joints is of paramount importance. This has been dealt with in Chapter 18. Check back on that. The points which need emphasis are:
1.   Do this work under the tuition and supervision of the hospital Physiotherapy Department, if possible. The standard routine is for the physiotherapists to instruct the relatives in the provision of this stimulus.
2.   The movements should be performed in reference to a joint chart, so that all joints which are accessible are dealt with.
3.   The programme of proprioceptive input is maintained during the whole of the coma-arousal programme, until spontaneous movement becomes established.
4.   It may be of value to provide combined movements of more than one limb. This may be done in a homolateral pattern initially, and then in a cross-pattern. (See Chapter 22.)
(Where there are lesions which affect joint work, for example, fractures, etc., movement of the limb may need to be withheld.)

Programme for Vestibular Stimulation

The programme for balance is dealt with in Chapter 18. Refer back to that. Remember that every change of head position is referred to our balance mechanisms. When we change our body position, we usually also change our head position and affect our sense of balance. Therefore to take patients from a lying position on the back and roll them over on their side is important. To sit them up is important. To take patients from the sitting position and place them face down on their hands and knees is important. To lift patients onto their knees is important. To stand them up is important. You will only do these things by degrees, not all at once. If you take the patient out in a wheelchair, he or she receives vestibular input. If you take them up and down in a lift, they receive balance input. Every movement of head and body is important.

This very important and primitive sense is often compromised in hospital by:

1.   Lying in bed for weeks or months;
2.   The effect of the brain injury on nerve and muscle function;

3. The use of drugs;
4. The use of inhibition plasters;
5. Other extracranial problems (e.g., fractures, chest problems).

The initial venture into anything related to balance and gravity can be very discomforting to the patient who has no control over his own body movement.

It is of paramount importance, therefore, that when any awareness has developed, none of these following manoeuvres should be performed initially without the presence of a relative who has the ability to calm and reassure the patient.

Since vestibular function is so dependent on movement of the head and body, it is of great importance that programmes should be arranged to provide this stimulation.

Briefly, the approach is:

1. Head movements should be undertaken within the range of the movement part of the programme. These movements should include flexion/extension, sideways tilting and rotation. There should also be opportunity for the patient's head to be placed below the level of the body for short periods of time.
2. The patient should be in the upright position as much as possible. The supine position is one of sleep, not arousal.
3. The patient should be placed upright on the edge of the bed with the feet overhanging, and rotated around that vertical pole.
4. The tilt table should be used for short periods as soon as the patient can safely cope with it.
5. As soon as is reasonable, the patient should be placed on a mat on the floor, and there rolling and rocking of the whole body should be provided.

CHAPTER 22

WHAT TO DO IN THE UNCONSCIOUS AND RESPONSIVE PATIENT — MOTOR OUTPUT

Before you read this chapter, you would be well advised to re-read Chapter 15, The Pathway of Recovery.

This book is only about coming out of coma. To include in detail the requirements for the regaining of movement would need another book. I will list, however, some of the methods which are available in rehabilitation facilities and which can even be set up relatively cheaply at home.

To arouse the patient from coma then, is only the first stage. To bring the patient to a point of arousal and then to leave them without any motor function, or with so little motor function that they are unable to do anything, is little gain to them or to anyone else. Motor function is of paramount importance.

MOTOR FUNCTIONS

	Limb and Body Movement	Hand Function	Vocalization
STAGE 1	No movement	No movement	No sound
STAGE 2	Reflex movement	Grasp reflex	Sounds
STAGE 3	Spontaneous movement	E.T. sign Hand release	Use of words
STAGE 4	Control of movement	Prehensile grasp	Use of sentences
STAGE 5	Fine control of movement	Pincer grasp	Correct conversation

The importance of movement

All movement is for survival or for reproduction. In our very primitive brain these two functions are absolute. Survival depends upon our abilities to find food or to control our relationship with an invader, either by fight or flight.

This ability to fight or flee depends upon four very important regions. These are:

1. Our head — which carries our reception and control centres. Our brain has a large component of our major senses and has the responsibility of positioning us in our environment.
2. Our body — which contains our vital organs such as heart, lungs, kidneys, bowels, etc., and which has the responsibility of performing all the vegetative functions.

The head and body constitute the main parts of the Central Axis.

3. Our legs which can move our body to a new environment and also provide a part of the Central Axis.
4. Our arms which can be used to protect our head and our body and which have those amazing objects called hands on the end of them.

We can live in an environment only when we can provide for our needs and protect ourselves, when we have these four areas working fully. We have a decreased ability to exist when specific areas fail to function. This is especially so when our head or body is injured and therefore the very centre of our physical being — our Central Axis — is affected.

It is possible to live without one leg. But the environment in which we move becomes more threatening as we have less ability to move our central axis out of danger. We can use tools and equipment to help transport us, but we are then very much dependent upon them or upon others to help.

Living without both legs is possible but the environment becomes even more threatening, since while it is possible to walk with a stick or crutch on one leg, such things are useless when both legs cannot function. Without legs, the only ways we may move our body are by rolling or by using our hands to pull us along face down like a snake or by sitting on our buttocks and swinging our weight on our hands and arms. None of these methods is strong or fast.

It is possible to live with only one arm but the ability to provide for, and protect, the central axis is decreased considerably. A one-armed person seeking food is considerably hampered, whether it is fishing, hunting, shooting, etc. In defence, one arm can only cover the head or the body, unlike the two-armed person who can use one arm to protect the head and the other to protect the body. Survival under assault becomes less certain for the one-armed man.

Our civilization judges people by what they can do — by their motor output or, in the term more familiar to us, by their performance.

Whether it is the Olympic Games or *The Barber of Seville* or a National Basketball game, the applause goes to the performers. Sensory function itself is judged by motor performance and rates very little in importance on its own. You may have the most acute eyesight or hearing or abilities to feel, taste or smell in the world but these abilities attract little attention if they are not made obvious by motor performance.

You, therefore, must pursue this regaining of the patient's ability to move with the utmost determination. Let nothing prevent you from attempting to achieve this goal.

Most severely brain-injured patients have problems with movement. These problems may be so severe that the patient is conscious, that is, awake and aware of the environment, but is unable to move head or arms or legs and is unable to talk. He/She is in what is called a "locked-in" state. (See Chapter 23) The only indication that the person is awake is that s/he may look towards you and even make eye contact. This must be the most terrible state to be in — to be aware and able to detect the stimuli of the environment but unable to respond in any meaningful way.

Many of these patients, both the vegetative patients and the locked in patients are not given the opportunity to regain their motor function. They are left in bed with a minimal amount of sensory input and the minimum opportunity to move. This negative approach to the severely brain-injured is a world-wide problem because of the attitude of the caring professions that these patients are Non People. I see this negative approach to be wrong and my opinion is shared by other people.

While it is acknowledged that some or many of the muscle movements outlined below may be compromised by the effect of the brain injury, this does not mean that they should not be sought. With correct help and the correct environment, some patients may be enabled to use their canalized processes and their intrinsic drive.

Probably the worst thing for the immobile patient is continuation of the immobility and while spontaneous movements must have returned before controlled movement can begin, the time taken to regain both spontaneous and controlled movements may be months or years.

The following is based on what is called the developmental approach. This really means that child development is used as a model for the restoring of motor function in the brain-injured person, whether child or adult. The functions are regained in a specific manner, much as the child develops abilities in a specific manner. Of course, as I have stressed before there is a difference in that the brain-injured person has already developed once through their childhood and the brain injury itself can affect the process of this redevelopment.

THE REGAINING OF MOTOR FUNCTION

Motor function seems to be regained in a sequential way.

STAGE 1	NO MOVEMENT
STAGE 2	REFLEX MOVEMENT
STAGE 3	SPONTANEOUS MOVEMENT
STAGE 4	CONTROLLED MOVEMENT
STAGE 5	FINE CONTROL OF MOVEMENT

MOTOR STAGE 1 AND STAGE 2

THE PATIENT *IN COMA* WITH NO MOVEMENT OR REFLEX MOVEMENT

When the patient is in coma and has no movement or has reflex movement the application of tactile stimuli to the total body surface is undertaken in an attempt to waken the patient and also to obtain reflex movement. At the same time in the programme, a passive range of movements should be used (i.e, you or someone else moving the limbs and body of the patient so that the joints will not stiffen and go into an abnormal position).

MOTOR STAGE 1 AND STAGE 2

THE PATIENT *OUT OF COMA* WITH NO MOVEMENT OR REFLEX MOVEMENT

When the patient is out of coma and has no movement the same procedure is followed — the regular application of stimuli to the face, arms, legs and body, always identifying where the stimulus is by speaking to the patient. Of course, the patient out of coma can also use his/her eyes and obtain visual information. Range of movement must be continued.

The same applies to the patient who has reflex movements. The stimuli should be maintained, seeking the reflex movement. Generally, these movements become stronger and with time need weaker stimuli to elicit them.

The big difference, however, is that the patient out of coma can usually understand what movement you want them to make and can co-operate in the striving to make it. It is of the utmost importance that at all times you should encourage and motivate the patient. Feed them only positives. Congratulate them when they have achieved, for their effort needs to be recognized and rewarded.

MOTOR STAGE 3 AND 4

THE PATIENT *OUT OF COMA* WITH SPONTANEOUS OR CONTROLLED MOVEMENT

Usually, constant work in attempting to obtain a reflex response to a stimulus will bring a reward. One day the patient will make a spontaneous movement of the head or arm or leg or body. This will very probably be of small size and very weak and apparently purposeless. Nevertheless, it is a major breakthrough for it implies that under certain conditions the brain has initiated a nerve impulse which has reached a muscle group and stimulated it to work. If those conditions can be repeated, then the movement may be repeated and not only repeated but become strengthened and constant.

While the movement may seem purposeless to us, to the patient it is an enormous breakthrough. For one instant, freedom is beckoning and can beckon again. We must applaud this breakthrough and encourage the whole process. It is quite unjustified for us to discount the effort by telling the patient that the movement is a coincidence — for us it may be a coincidence but for the patient it may be a reward for effort.

With time, effort, practice, motivation, love, encouragement, demand by the relatives, friends, therapists and positive feed back to the patient, it is hoped that the spontaneous movement will one day come within the control of the patient. Again, this control will be slowly established, perhaps taking months or years to reach good function.

With all of the movements it is important to give the patient a goal to aim for. Do not make it too difficult. Make it achievable. It might be to move a part of the body or a limb to a certain mark. If it is not achieved, reduce the difficulty of the goal so that it can be achieved. When it is obtained, pour out your congratulations.

Breathing also is tremendously important. Get the patient to take a deep breath before each movement.

The Areas to be Worked

There are four major components which need to be identified and worked on in an attempt to regain motor output. These have been alluded to in the beginning of this chapter.

These are;

1 THE CENTRAL AXIS — THE CONTROL OF THE HEAD
2 THE CENTRAL AXIS — THE STATIONARY CONTROL OF THE BODY
3 THE CENTRAL AXIS — MOVING THE AXIS — THE LEGS
4 THE CENTRAL AXIS — PROTECTING THE AXIS — THE ARMS

THE IMPORTANCE OF THE CENTRAL AXIS

By the Central Axis I mean the vertical component of our person i.e., our head, neck and body. You will recall in Chapter 12, I wrote about motor function in terms of a gun emplacement and how important it is for the gun to have a firm and stable base. It is the same with our bodies. We depend upon the Central Axis to be the base from which we move our arms to provide manual competence and our legs to provide mobility. It is, therefore, of the greatest importance to seek and obtain a patient who can at least hold his or her head upright in a balanced position and who can also maintain a sitting position.

I will list some of the methods used in an attempt to restore the most important functions.

1 THE CENTRAL AXIS — THE CONTROL OF THE HEAD

The ability to control the head is of enormous importance. Often you will find that the patient is unable to lift his/her head upright but can balance it for a short time if it is placed there.

The Position of Balance

Even for the patient merely to have the head held up in the mid position and then attempt to balance it, is of benefit. If necessary, help the patient to hold up the head and then place your hand on the top to stabilize it. At first, the patient may only be able to hold up his/her head with a great deal of support, but after practice you may be able to help him or her maintain position just by holding the hair. Often s/he will need some support behind the head and while initially this needs to be something soft and comfortable, after progress is made, a firm surface may be better.

Sometimes it is worth putting on a neck collar to provide some support but only do this for, say, periods of 30 minutes at a time.

Always try to stop the head falling forward with a jolt. Keep your hands close, so that when it does begin to fall, you can support it.

The Rotation of the Head

You want the person to be able to turn their head in both directions, that is towards either shoulder. It is highly unlikely that they will be able to do this at first, but keep putting yourself or other interesting people and things to the side which is weakest and invite the patient to turn the head towards you or the object. Often it is worthwhile so placing the bed in the room that the patient is forced to turn the head towards the door where most of the interesting events are occurring. Also place the TV set so the patient must turn towards it. It is a good idea to vary its position each day.

The Elevation of the Head

Lifting the head is also of great importance. This seems to be very slow to come in some patients, because the head does weigh so much and the muscles necessary to pull it up are often very weak.

When this lifting movement becomes stronger it is worthwhile placing the patient on the floor in the face down position. You know the typical baby picture with the baby on its stomach lifting its head. This is the same position. Sometimes, the lifting of the head is easier if the patient is on a balloon or bolster which already supports the shoulders.

2 THE CENTRAL AXIS — THE CONTROL OF THE BODY

The Tilt Table

All hospitals which deal with severe brain injury have a tilt table. This is a table on which the patient lies, strapped in safely with three broad straps, which is tilted slowly, raising the head so the patient can eventually be placed upright with the feet on a small platform at the bottom.

This table is of enormous importance. Not only does it allow the patient to come into the upright position, which is a position of awareness; it also changes the stresses on the different muscles, bones and joints and brings them into a more normal state. Also it has a marked effect on the heart and blood vessels, reducing the pooling of blood and tissue fluid in the back of the body and bringing it back into circulation. The lungs also benefit. The diaphragm drops with the aid of gravity when the patient is upright, and the pressure of the contents of the abdomen is taken off it and the lungs can expand.

There are, of course, some precautions to be taken. The process of elevation should be gradual and for the first few days, the angle of elevation may only be 20-30 degrees. It is important also to watch the breathing of the patient and make routine checks of the blood pressure so that fainting does not occur.

Returning the patient to the horizontal should also be done slowly and the patient observed. In fact, it is a learning experience for you to try the tilt table to feel what it is like.

The Sit Up

Often, because of weakness of the trunk muscles, the patient has difficulty in sitting up. This can be seen fairly early after the brain injury when the patient is placed in a chair and needs many pillows to prop him or her up. Usually with time, the tone or resting muscle power of the body improves and the patient tries to sit up or can help in the process of being sat up. One way to help the patient gain more control is to reduce the number of pillows provided for support in the chair, ensure that the chair has arm rests and is fairly hard backed. By this, I do not mean to make the patient uncomfortable. Reduce the number of pillows gradually in relation to the patient's improving ability to sit up. The time variation in abilities of these patients must always be at the forefront of your mind and you must be aware that on some days patients will not cope so well, whereas on other days, you will be pleasantly surprised by their performance.

The Bed Edge

When the patient is strong enough, it is worthwhile sitting him or her on the edge of the bed with legs hanging over the edge. Initially, s/he may need a great deal of support at the back and also on each side. You may have to get on to the bed, kneeling behind the patient, to give this back support. While you do, encourage the patient to sit up. If s/he is not doing well, just provide a short time in this position. If all is going well talk to him or her about how strong s/he is becoming and how well she or he is doing. Feed your positives to them.

You will usually find, as the days and weeks and months pass, power to sit up will return.

The Small Bolster

One other method to start to obtain body control, especially if the patient has trouble maintaining a sitting position, is to place them front down over a round bolster about 18 inches (45 cm) high. Put the hands on the floor at the front and the feet on the floor at the back and see if they can control their body while it is supported on the bolster. If they are very weak, it may be necessary to provide some support by placing a controlling hand on their back or by holding on to their bottom.

The Quadriped Position

When they have strengthened, it is worthwhile trying the person in a quadriped position (i.e., on all fours like a dog or horse). They may not be able to maintain this position at first and it is worthwhile, if you are strong enough, straddling them and looping your arms around their chest or abdomen to give them support. After they gain strength you can place a small padded stool in front of them and place the arms on this. You can also place them with the elbows down on the floor, which will help them to become stronger.

Always make sure that you have enough people around to support the patient so s/he will not become worried.

The Knee Stand

To move into a knee stand or the praying position is always a great venture. It implies that the body has enough strength to hold itself upright with support if necessary. The best piece of equipment to use is a small table with a centre part cut out so the chest can be set into the table. Don't worry if you do not have this however. The essential thing is to have a comfortable and solid piece of furniture such as a heavy chair which will not move forward when you place the front of the patient's body against the back of the chair. Put the patient on his/her knees and hook the arms over the top of the chair. At first they may complain of back pain. Usually if you ask them if they can put up with it for a few minutes they will. If they cannot, then it is obviously wise to have their spine checked.

The Exercise Bicycle

Once control comes, it is worthwhile using an exercise bicycle and placing their feet in the pedals, supporting them while in this position and seeing if they can strengthen up. Do not be worried about getting them to attempt to pedal, although if they wish to try, do not discourage them.

The Wall Stand

If the person is able to take some weight on one or both legs, place them in the corner between two walls, if necessary supporting them on each side at first. You may only be able to leave them for a few minutes or even less, depending upon how they feel. Day by day, strength will come.

Often you will note that the feet become swollen. This is natural with the change in position but if you are worried ask the physician to check.

3 THE CENTRAL AXIS — MOVING THE AXIS — THE LEGS

One of the most comfortable pieces of furniture yet devised is the bean bag. Sitting in it, a person can burrow in, but even for a person with good motor abilities it can be difficult to push up and get out. For the person with motor disability, the bean bag can be a disaster. Every movement is yielded to by the soft beans. There is virtually no resistance. The chance of shifting position becomes even more difficult and the fight to change position dies. In many ways, the patient is now reminiscent of the beetle on its back, stuck and unable to move the central axis.

The Roll

When the patient is lying on the mat, if they have some leg movement, they may be able to roll from their back on to their side. Often this is easier to do when they roll on to their weakest side, rolling their good leg over the other leg first and then twisting their body. If they are not able to do this, it is worthwhile lying them on their side and encouraging them to move so they roll on to the front of their body.

The Ability to Move the Legs

Often the patient will move one or both legs. They can do this while lying in bed, but sometimes they find it easier to do while sitting on the edge of the bed or in a chair where the effects of gravity can be a help. As they become stronger, it is possible to sit them in a wheel-chair and ask them to push away from you, and to pull themselves to you, while you sit in front and hold their feet or ankles.

Raising the Buttocks

Many patients strengthen both their body and their legs by lying on their back and elevating their bottom off the mat. Sometimes it is necessary to hold the feet to provide stability while this exercise is being done.

Patterning

Much work on patterning has been done by The Institutes for The Achievement of Human Potential in Philadelphia and reference is made to Chapter 11 in Glenn Doman's book *What To Do About Your Brain Injured Child* (Doubleday and Company, Inc. Garden City, New York 1974). Chapter 13 in Ian Hunter's book *Brain Injury* (Hill of Content, Australia, 1986) also gives a good insight into patterning.

Patterning is an attempt to put primitive movements of head, body, arms and legs into the brain by passive movement. Basically there are two major patterns, both of them quite simple — the *homolateral* and the *crossed* pattern.

With both types of pattern the patient lies face down on a padded bench at waist height of the five helpers — one at the head and one at each of the limbs. In the homolateral pattern the patient's head is turned from the midline position to the right while the right arm is brought forward very much like a swimming stroke until the wrist is as far forward as the hair on the head. At the same time, the right leg is moved; the heel first being pushed down inside towards the bench with the patterners left hand and her right hand being placed behind the patient's knee. The leg is then pushed towards the front of the bench thus bending the leg forward at the hip and knee. The head is then moved to the left, while the right arm and leg are taken back, the left arm and leg are taken forward. The pattern then continues for a period of minutes.

The *crossed* pattern is very similar. The only difference is that when the head is turned to the right, and while the right arm goes forward, it is the left leg which is moved. Conversely when the head is turned to the left and looks towards the left arm, it is the right leg which is brought forward.

These patterns have been used by us with good effect. Certainly the patients appear to wake up while this movement is going on and we also notice that while their muscles may be very tight or contracted to begin with, they tend to loosen. At the present level of our experience, it is impossible to say more about patterning.

The Slide

Man has a built-in demand to move, and this demand is to move forward. Our eyes face forward — our bodies move forward. If we are not able to walk or crawl forwards, we may still be able to slide forward by pushing and pulling. With a slide board about one metre wide and about five metres long, smooth and powdered, strong enough to support the weight of the patient, elevated at the top end to about 30 or 40 degrees, it may be possible to get the patient to slide.

Obviously the angle of inclination needs to be suitable for the patient and the patient needs to be surrounded by caring, loving people. She or he is placed on the board face down with a towel under the face and encouraged to wriggle down the board using whatever methods are feasible. If possible, the arms are used to pull and the legs to push, often with a helper's hand to stabilise the pushing foot.

Crawling

When the patient becomes strong enough to maintain the quadriped position, it is worthwhile asking them if they would like to try to crawl. They may need knee pads and you should make sure that the surface is carpeted and reasonably soft. If they do wish to crawl, insist that they move very slowly and only move one limb at a time. See if you can get them to do a *homolateral* crawl first, turning the head to the right, bringing the right arm forward and then the right leg. Then turn the head to the left, bring up the left arm and then the left leg and continue on in this way.

When they have mastered this pattern, move on to the *crossed pattern* with the head turning to the right, the right arm being brought forward and then the left leg. The next move is obviously to turn the head to the left, bring up the left arm and then the right leg and continue on in this way.

The Knee Crawl

When the patient is strong enough in the knee stand position, it is time to start the knee crawl. Place the patient on his or her knees with arms forward and hands on the shoulders of a person kneeling facing them. While the helper moves back, the patient slowly moves forward.

Walking

How everyone wants to walk! We all recognise walking as one of our primitive instincts. When the corner stand is strong and the crawling is strong, it is time to consider the walk. Often people find it easier to walk with a walking frame, but if this is not available, it is a good idea just to cruise around a wall. If you can find one with a handrail so much the better. Have the patient balance and very slowly move parallel with the wall, while holding the handrail or forward using the walking frame.

The technique of *Brachiation*, developed by the Institutes of Human Potential is also important. With a ladder suspended above the head of the patient, at a height which they can easily reach, the patient is encouraged to walk along with arms outstretched and hands clasping the bars and supporting some of their weight.

214

4 THE CENTRAL AXIS — PROTECTING THE AXIS — THE ARMS

Our arms protect our central axis to a distance of an arm's length to the front and out to the sides and even towards the back. We swing them like boxers protecting our personal space. With coarse weapons such as bayonets and swords we extend our protective distance. With finer tools such as slings, boomerangs, bows and arrows, spears and guns we extend our protected distance still further.

Passive Arm Movements

The importance of moving the arms, even if there are no spontaneous movements, has been dealt with before. Do not allow the arms to fix. Sit the patient up if possible. Use a wooden rod about the thickness of a broom handle as this is a good working tool and easily obtainable. Usually patients do have a grasp reflex and it is worth inserting the rod into their hands while they are upright on the tilt table, with you facing them, your hands on the rod and using the rod to pull the patient's arms up and down and around, even twisting as if to go around a clock face.

Active Arm Movements

The arms of the brain-injured person usually, but not always, tend to be bent at the elbows and resting across the chest or abdomen. They frequently have some movement across these two areas. The most important part our hands move to, and the movement which has the most practice normally is to our mouth. Even in infants, the major movement of the hand is to the mouth and you will all no doubt recall seeing infants placing everything into their mouths.

Since this is such a built-in movement, it is worth using as much as possible. While the patient may not be able to grasp a spoon, it is possible to provide an instrument which may allow the patient to feed himself or herself. What we often do is place some playdough in a wide 20 ml capacity syringe, push the wooden or plastic handle of a flavoured ice block into the dough and put the wide tube of the syringe into the hands of the patient.

Equipment

The use of weights of varying size, gymnasium equipment, massage, heat, biofeedback machines are all important and should be used when warranted.

This sequential regaining of mobility should be undertaken in a work-like manner.

Hand function

It is wise to seek out the services of an Occupational Therapist to help with hand function.

THE FIVE STAGES OF MANUAL COMPETENCE.

STAGE 1	NO REACTION TO STIMULUS
STAGE 2	THE GRASP REFLEX

STAGE 3	GRASP RELEASE
STAGE 4	PREHENSILE GRASP
STAGE 5	PINCER GRASP

Anyone who cannot demonstrate manual competence is at a grave disadvantage. Survival in a primitive society is dependent on the ability to use the hands for hunting, agriculture and defence (weapons, etc.). The person in our culture who cannot use his hands for writing, manipulation of tools, etc., is also in a state of disadvantage.

The Grasp Reflex

The grasp reflex often tends to return even in those who initially had no grasp. Working the hand passively, flexing and extending all the fingers and thumb many times every day is very important.

The Grasp Release

Constantly placing objects, especially your hand, into that of the patient and asking him or her to let go may help to bring about a better release mechanism. Sometimes if they will not let go it is helpful to exert some heavy pressure on to the web between the thumb and first finger in an effort to secure release.

When these functions have returned it is worthwhile challenging the grasp regularly every day in an endeavour to improve grasp and release.

The Prehensile Grasp

Once controlled grasp and release are present, constantly seeking the grasp action by giving objects to the patient to pick up will help to obtain better grasp. Initially, the object may be held by the palm with little control by the fingers but eventually the power and control of the fingers may return.

The Pincer Grasp

The ability to hold an object between finger and thumb is one of the hallmarks of the human. Constant practice by giving objects to the patient to grasp between the finger and thumb is needed.

Speech

The advice of a sympathetic Speech Therapy Department may be of great assistance.

Speech is an undoubted indicator of cortical function. Re-development of speech is sequential but is severely compromised by the site and extent of the brain injury. It is also prevented by the continuing presence of a tracheostomy and affected by the presence of a naso-gastric tube.

The first noise which the patient makes is likely to be in response to discomfort or to an emotional episode.

It is possible that application of touch, ice, etc., to the lips, mouth and tongue may help to re-establish the mechanisms of speech. There appear to be precursors of speech such as clicking of the tongue, sucking sounds and attempted mouthing of words.

The patient will often make incomprehensible sounds which can be quite grotesque, but this may be the only method of communication which she or he has. It should therefore be treated with the same respect which is accorded to any other person and every effort should be made to try to understand what the patient wishes to say.

Speech is also often accompanied by some body movement which also should be respected as body language. This may include crying and other signs of distress. When speech does return, it is also frequently in response to some discomfort or to an emotional situation.

Talking and reading to the patient should be viewed as an essential part of any programme.

Feeding

The advice of a sympathetic Occupational Therapist is invaluable.

Feeding is obviously a very primitive behaviour. Like all primitive behaviours, it is canalized and there is an intrinsic drive that it should be fulfilled by a natural method.

Naso-gastric tubes should not be used for longer than is necessary. The longer a patient remains on artificial feeding, the more remote becomes his or her independence.

In many patients it may be possible to provide oral feeding weeks and months before it is believed possible. There are a number of reasons for the delay.

These are;

1. The patient is seen as being still life-threatened when this is not so.
2. There is the real worry of fluid and food being drawn into the lungs. This can cause pneumonia and threaten the life of the patient.
3. There is inadequate trust between the person providing the food and the patient.
4. Insufficient time is allowed for the feeding.
5. The food offered is not acceptable to the patient. i.e., cold, poor taste, food which the patient customarily dislikes.

I would therefore suggest that;

1. Patients should be fed orally as soon as is possible. This should not only depend on the customary weekly assessments but should be at the request of those most in touch with the patients, i.e., the relatives.
2. Relatives should be properly taught how to feed the patient, and should do so under supervision, initially at least.
3. They should be warned that this is a time-consuming business and should allow sufficient time for the feeding.

4. They should be in a state of harmony with the patient.
5. The food should be offered to the patient on one of his or her "good" days.
6. The appropriate food which is basically to the patient's liking should be offered, if possible, in a manner to which s/he is accustomed and in a way which s/he likes.
7. Failure at one time should be viewed as temporary and a determined effort made to set up the best conditions for another attempt as soon as possible.

Conclusion

Respect for the patient, hard work, consistency, love are the bastions upon which the return of motor function depends. The time of recovery is prolonged. No one can yet say how long or how successful it will be. But it is worth the effort.

PROLONGED COMA

CHAPTER 23   PROLONGED COMA —
PERSISTENT VEGETATIVE STATE —
THE LOCKED-IN STATE

CHAPTER 23

PROLONGED COMA — PERSISTENT VEGETATIVE

STATE — THE LOCKED-IN STATE

There are three states of coma, or comalike state, which need to be dealt with in some detail and separately. They have very great repercussions for the patient and the family and the community. They are prolonged coma, the persistent vegetative state and the locked-in state.

1. Prolonged Coma

The severity of a brain injury is measured by both the depth and duration of coma: that is, how deep is it and how long does it last. On the international assessment using the Glasgow Coma Scale (see Chapter 2), a person in coma for six hours or longer is regarded as having a severe brain injury. If the patient remains in coma for two weeks or longer, then they are said to be in prolonged coma.

The results of prolonged coma, according to information available at this time, appear to be very poor. One person who has investigated prolonged coma from trauma, is Dr A. Bricolo. He and his colleagues, wrote on this topic in the *Journal of Neurosurgery*, 52: 625-634, 1980, an article entitled "Prolonged post-traumatic unconsciousness". He and his colleagues looked at post-traumatic coma in 135 patients. These patients may not all have been in coma, for the classification of the patients was made on the basis that the patients were either unresponsive two weeks after the onset of coma, or incapable of executing simple commands, or showing any rapport with their environment.

His results showed that at the end of one year:

30%	died
8%	survived in a vegetative state
31%	survived with severe disabilities
18%	had moderate disability
13%	had a good recovery

These results would indicate that prolonged coma is a very serious problem, and that every effort should be made to arouse the patient from coma as soon as possible.

2. The Persistent Vegetative State

When prolonged coma continues for months, the patient is classified as being in the Persistent Vegetative State (PVS). The actual point of time at which this diagnosis is made varies. It depends upon the surgeon, the country, the age of the patient, and the relatives.

Many authorities consider that a patient still in coma at three months after the trauma is in the persistent vegetative state (PVS). Other authorities consider that six months is a more correct time at which to apply the label.

No matter what the time-frame, the implications are enormous for the patient. If the results are so poor with patients in prolonged coma for two weeks, the prognosis for patients in coma for months must be seen as worse. The diagnosis virtually means that there is no hope of achieving anything with the patient, and that they will be placed in a care situation without any real attempt to arouse or restore function. I asked the director of a rehabilitation unit what he did with the patients in persistent vegetative state. His reply was "We store them in A ward." When I then asked who looked after them, he replied, "No one. What is the use?"

In some countries I have visited, when I have enquired about the management of the persistent vegetative state, I have been told that they do not have such patients. When I have expressed amazement at this statement, I have been told that after two weeks in coma, maintenance and resuscitative measures have been ceased.

Professor A.G.M. Campbell, Professor of Child Health at the University of Aberdeen, Scotland, writing in the *British Medical Journal*, Vol. 289, p.1022, makes the statement that PVS is a "fate worse than death". He writes PVS "describes those patients with irreversible brain damage . . . and who on recovery from deep coma pass into a state of seeming wakefulness and reflex responsiveness, but do not return to a cognitive sapient state." This brings us to the definition of this state.

Definition of Persistent Vegetative State

The persistent vegetative state was initially defined by Jennett and Plum in the medical journal, *The Lancet* (1972, April 1). They considered that, "It is the discrepancy between prolonged periods of wakefulness and the absence of any behavioural or physiological evidence of cortical function or mental activity, which characterises the vegetative state."

Really, what they were saying was that the eyes of the patient were usually open for periods of the day, giving the appearance of wakefulness, but that the patient showed no evidence that he or she had an awareness of their own person or of the environment or could think. The patient is awake, but *not aware*.

The essential component, according to Jennett and Plum, is "The absence of any adaptive response to the external environment, the absence of any evidence of a functioning mind which is either receiving or projecting information, in a patient who has long periods of wakefulness."

The words, "absence of any adaptive response to the external environment", really are saying that no one has seen the patient attempt to "do" anything to change their environment. Because no one has seen the patient "do" anything, then the supposition is made that the mind is incapable of taking in information or of giving out information. (You will recall in previous chapters how the mind is really an information-processing organ.)

In diagrammatic form this state is

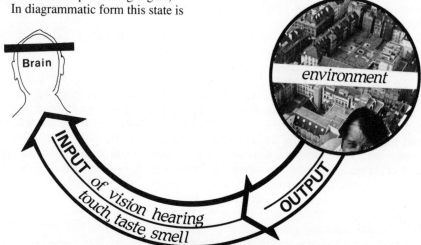

Figure 23.1. The Persistent Vegetative State

Dr F. Plum and Dr J. Posner in their book, *The Diagnosis of Stupor and Coma* (F.A.Davis and Co., Philadelphia 1980) see the patient as having no "outward manifestations of higher mental activity".

The Incidence of PVS

The incidence of PVS varies from study to study. A frequently used figure is that approximately 4 per cent of all severe brain injuries go into the vegetative state. It may be assumed that more and more of these patients, who previously would have died, have survived over the last ten to fifteen years, due to the improvement in the rapid resuscitation and transit of the patient to the hospital, the improvement in the accident and emergency care, the rapid diagnosis and operative procedures, and the great improvements in the intensive care units.

Is it possible to identify PVS accurately?

A review of the relevant medical publications suggests that it is possible to identify PVS with reasonable certainty by expert serial neuro assessment of the coma, in addition to the clinical methods of assessment of the patient at the bedside. The profession now depends heavily upon detecting the brain waves by Electroencephalograms (EEG), the use of a measure of the input of stimuli to the brain by Evoked Potentials (EP), X-rays of the brain with Computerized Tomography (CT) and with the newly developed diagnostic tool, the Nuclear Magnetic Resonance machine (NMR).

It is important to ask how accurate are these diagnostic tools separately, and in unison, and to determine if they have the ultimate proven right to be the decision-makers in such a life-and-death situation, or are there other sources of information which can be brought to bear on the problem.

It has been noted that the relatives frequently disagree with the diagnosis of persistent vegetative state. Bricolo and his colleagues (1980) noted this fact when they wrote, "There always remains the lingering doubt that the patient may in fact have some mental activity which we have simply failed to detect." He points to those caring for the patient, as often having a contrary view to the doctor when he says, " . . . this doubt is often kindled by claims from those caring for the vegetative wreck on a fulltime basis that the patient actually makes himself understood in some uncommon or even eerie way."

Jennett and Plum (1972) recognized the difficulty of establishing the diagnosis when they conceded that the judgment was made on the observation of behaviour of the patient and stated that "this concept may be criticized on the grounds that observation of behaviour is insufficient evidence on which to base a judgment of mental activity." But they wrote, "There is no reliable alternative available to the doctor at the bedside, which is where the decisions have to be made."

This statement was made before the development of many of the sophisticated measures of assessment just outlined. Since the new tools have not, however, been tested for a sufficiently long period of time in making the diagnosis of the persistent vegetative state, their accuracy is yet to be decided.

Often, what also happens is that the diagnosis is "muddled". The doctor is really unsure of what is happening to the patient. There is no doubt about the severity of the brain injury, and there appears to be no evidence of a thinking brain, but the doctor is reluctant to use the words, persistent vegetative state. No real diagnosis is made, but the patient is put down as "beyond rehabilitation".

Gail Graham, in her book *Staying Alive* (Angus and Robertson, Sydney, 1985), tells of the experiences of her son Jimmy, who was thought to be vegetative. Years after the accident he was able to use a pointing board on to which he spelt out, "kill me."

The *New York Times*, in its magazine section of June 1982 has an article entitled "Coming Out of Coma", which details cases of patients in the persistent vegetative state who have emerged from coma at prolonged periods of time from the accident.

Professor A.G.M. Campbell has concerns also. He says, "For children especially, a minimum period of three months seems prudent before they are deemed to be permanently unconscious" and "Children in coma are more unpredictable than adults . . . this uncertainty should make us particularly cautious in making hasty judgments about prognosis" and "No matter how carefully the medical criteria are selected, and no matter how accurate they are in predicting outcome, there will always be some uncertainty." He also says, "Recovery is rare in patients who have been in the vegetative state for one month."

Doubts about the diagnosis are also raised if the relatives are at variance with the professional opinions.

While it is possible the relatives may indulge in wishful thinking, this has not been the case in the relatives of 14 persistent vegetative state patients surveyed. In the majority of cases, verification of the opinions of the relatives was obtained from senior nursing or paramedical staff.

All of the patients were six months or more from the time of brain insult. Three of the patients were in a general hospital, one was in a district hospital, one in a rehabilitation hospital, two in psychiatric hospitals, three in a nursing home and four in terminal care.

The age range was from 17 years old to 45 years old. Six of the patients were under 20 years old, five were between 20 and 30 years old, two were 30 to 40 years old and one over 40 years old.

Ten of the 14 patients had sustained a traumatic brain injury in a road accident.

Questions which were asked of the relatives and staff to establish behavioural responses were:

1. Do you think the patient knows if someone is present?
2. Does the patient react differently depending upon who is present?
3. Does the patient react differently to a changed environment?

Confirmation was sought as to the frequency of this response and if the observation had been made by more than one person. In regard to every patient, the answers to the questions asked above were positive.

Facial changes of expression were then sought on the basis that there is a link between emotion and cognition. Questions asked were related to those emotional facial changes defined by C. Izard (*Measuring Emotions in Infants and Children*, Cambridge University Press, 1982):

4. Are there facial changes of:
   anxiety, fear, anger, sadness, disgust, contempt, surprise, pleasure?

In 13 of the 14 groups asked, the answer was affirmative. Information was sought to see if the emotional facial change was appropriate to the circumstances, and in the majority this appeared to be the case.

5. Any evidence of independence of action was sought, no matter how minute, by asking relatives and staff if they felt that the patient co-operated or resisted in any way.

In 13 of the 14 groups asked, the answer was positive.

While evidence of this nature must be regarded as "soft", to diagnose a patient as being vegetative, mindless, and having no mental activity, when that being has evidence of awareness, is to confirm the incarceration of a mind inside a non-functioning body.

If this does occur, this presents a major moral and ethical dilemma for the relatives, the profession and the community.

The Effect of the Diagnosis of PVS

On the Patient

If the diagnosis is inaccurate, the effect on the patient is catastrophic. If he or she is capable of receiving stimuli, but not transmitting a motor action, and is regarded as a non-sentient being (that is, regarded as a "thing", a "non-person"), the psychological effects must be assumed to be devastating. Obviously, some patients close down their autonomic nervous system and wither away. Others must live in the hope that someone will recognize their plight and attempt to help them.

On the Relatives

Relatives who insist that the patient has an awareness are very vulnerable to the medical profession. They are seen initially as unrealistic and either refusing or incapable of accepting reality. Usually, they have prolonged periods of time with a social worker who attempts to get them to accept the reality of the diagnosis of the patient and their own situation. They are told to "go away and forget the problem", or, "go and live a new life," both of which most people find themselves totally incapable of doing. They still love the patient, still see him or her as a person. They realize how vulnerable that person is in a system which appears not to care enough and wishes to discard, or store, or warehouse the patient. They now see that the system, finding them an embarrassment, wishes them to abdicate from the position of close relationship and abandon the patient.

If this effort fails, the system, inadvertently or sometimes deliberately, convinced that it is correct in its judgment, commences to divide and separate the relatives. The husband or wife, whichever appears to be most stable to the patient's adviser, is drawn aside for a separate interview, and either a direct statement or an inference is made that the one who is most opposed to accepting the diagnosis, is becoming mentally and emotionally unstable. If this relative is receptive, he or she is urged to support the established medical opinion and to attempt to get the erring relative "to see reason". Having split the family support structure, it is relatively easy to label the relative who is reluctant to accept the diagnosis as needing psychiatric help.

This may lead to medication (= use of drugs) or institutionalization of a family member, weakening the family support structure, and compounding the whole problem.

On the Profession

All the professionals involved with the management of severe brain injury are committed to looking after many other patients. Just as the child who does well at school tends to receive more from the teacher, so does the patient who is doing well in hospital receive more from the staff.

Acute Hospitals, quite rightly, run with a rapid turnover of patients. They are geared to the patient who will get better, at least for a while. Unless there is a flow of patients out, the whole system becomes stagnant. Brain-injured patients clog up the system for months. Medical administrators need to keep the flow going. Therefore, at the very highest administrative level, the long-term patient who is unknown, except for a medical record number, is seen as a burden on the hospital services and a patient to be off-loaded as soon as possible. The attending physician is also in a difficult position. He or she has no therapy to offer to the patient, and he or she is aware that this soon becomes obvious to the relatives. The physician is caught in a cleft stick with a patient for whom nothing apparently can be done.

One approach to the problem patient is that taken by Professor Campbell, who writes, "I believe that anything, including feeding, that prolongs this non-human or artificial life is wrong for the child, wrong for the family, wrong for society", and many would agree with him.

In general, the attitude in the nursing staff and paramedicals changes when there appears to be no improvement in the patient's condition over weeks and months. If the patient is incapable of talking or giving any feedback, the patient is considered to be incapable of receiving or responding to stimuli, and therefore as a non-sentient, non-person, non-being.

How the System Deals with the PVS Patient

If Professor Campbell's management is not acceptable, the patient remains a problem. Patients in PVS may survive almost a normal lifespan, as long as adequate nutrition, nursing and control of infection is provided. Dr E.Le Winn, in his book *Coma Arousal: The Family as a Team* (The Better Baby Press, Philadephia, 1982) writes of a unit in the USA where it is anticipated that a 20-year-old comatose patient can be kept alive, still comatose, for fifty years.

There is, therefore, an intense drive to get the patient out of the acute hospital. Some are sent to terminal-care hospitals — hospices for the dying being used for patients who are not dying. Others are sent to nursing homes where they tend to have a variety of nursing care, varying from extremely good to very poor. Others are taken home to be looked after by their relatives with the help of community nurses and friends.

Another, more modern approach was presented at the International Conference on Health, Law and Ethics in Sydney, 1986. Professor David Smith, from the Vanderbilt University School of Law, Tennessee, suggested that patients in the persistent vegetative state should have life terminated at surgically convenient transplantation times, so they could become a source of organ donations. The words used for this approach are "to harvest the organs of the patients". The term "neomorts" has been coined for these patients. The rough estimate is that there are almost 10,000 patients in the USA who come within the category of neomorts.

Before Professor Smith's suggestion could even be contemplated, the diagnosis of the patient in the persistent vegetative state, as truly vegetative, would need to be absolute.

The extensive discussion at this particular conference on the ethical importance of prolonged coma indicates that this state presents a major moral and ethical dilemma for the relatives, the profession and the community and constitutes a field for further research.

What Should be the Approach to the Patient in PVS

Obviously, aspects of the diagnosis and management of the patient in PVS are unsatisfactory and unacceptable to many people. These two aspects, diagnosis and management, need to be clarified.

The Diagnosis

If the final judgment of a terminal condition is to be made on behavioural grounds at the bedside, both the judge should be defined and so should the behavioural grounds.

At present there are two parties who judge, often reaching different conclusions: the relatives and the doctors.

Merging the knowledge into a common arena may be of benefit to all, since the relatives, knowing the thinking and mannerisms of the patient and spending much time at the bedside, are admirably placed to give an opinion on the mental state of the patient.

It would, therefore, seem appropriate that the relatives and other providers of care, should be consulted by the doctors to determine if, from a behavioural viewpoint, a patient is responding in a meaningful way.

The behavioural grounds need to be clarified. Obviously the whole of the diagnosis hangs on the identification of *awareness*. The patient who is aware cannot be declared vegetative. Therefore, every sign of awareness must be sought and identified. This is a field of research, and the profession must recognize that the relatives have a right to be information-seekers.

Difficulties do arise where the signs of awareness are so fleeting and fragile that they are difficult to duplicate and present in a confirmed form. The use of video cameras as a monitoring system may be a solution to this problem. The other major factor will need to be an open and receptive mind by the professional, since the relatives are so vulnerable to a hostile environment provided by the "experts".

The Management — A Trial Of Arousal

Professor Campbell is in agreement with the approach which I believe to be correct, although it would appear that he would not provide such an intense or prolonged effort at arousal as I believe necessary. He writes, "Every opportunity should be taken to enrich the child's environment for maximum stimulation and to *identify signs of awareness*. Tapes of favourite voices and music should be available. Family members should be encouraged to participate in ways that may allow them to face the future realistically and help them in working out their grief."

Once again we come back to the pioneering work of Dr Le Winn and Dr Dimancescu, in an article on coma printed in *The Lancet* in 1978 (Vol. 2: 156), where they detailed their results in patients provided with coma arousal soon after trauma.

The techniques outlined in the section THE THERAPY should be carried out for a period of three months to see if any gain can be achieved.

It is essential:

1. To video the patient before the trial commences, so that a true record can be established for future reference.
2. To ensure that the programme is provided in a correct fashion, both in quantity and quality.
3. To document the changes as fully as possible.

4. To be aware that this is a full-time work, which, once embarked on, should only be reviewed at the correct time, unless there are severe contraindications.
5. To understand that no guarantee can be given for a successful outcome.
6. To know that it is only when the patient is aroused from coma that the true state of the injury becomes obvious.
7. To be aware that the patient out of coma with severe disability will need to be placed on to another programme to restore function, once again with these first five conditions applying.

At the end of three months, with an open mind and with a spirit of enquiry and with the questionnaire from Chapter 9 completed and with the videos, a meeting should be held with the medical and nursing and paramedical staff and the decision made on all available material as to the continuance or discontinuance of the programme.

Medicine is constantly working on trials of procedures or drug therapy, etc., and this approach should be acceptable to most orthodox practitioners.

In my own experience I recall two young men, both consigned to a terminal-care hospital. One, F.R., was given an intensive input of sensory and motor rehabilitation for a period of some months in the terminal-care facility, during which time he slowly improved to the point where his physician rang me up to say that the patient was "too good for terminal care" and was being transferred to a hospital for rehabilitation. He has since returned home.

The other patient, S.R., also in a hospice for the dying, having been declared vegetative after six months in a major university hospital, was closely examined. After the examination I told his parents that I felt that their son was not vegetative, and that certainly for some periods of time their son was out of coma. This was totally contrary to the earlier diagnosis which had been given to them. They had been told since early in the post-accident period that their son would be a vegetable and that nothing could be done to help him. He lay in that teaching hospital for six months, waiting to see if there would be any change, but when it became evident that there was no noticeable improvement, he was transferred to a hospice for the dying.

When I explained to the parents that I thought their son had indications that he was not in coma, they had some trouble believing the statement, but as I pointed out to them in a commonsense way what I had found, they began to understand. I asked them the standard questions (in Chapter 9) relating to vigilance, and back came the answers in the affirmative. "Yes," they did think that their son knew if they were present or not. "Yes," they did think that he reacted differently to different people. "Yes," they thought he reacted when he was placed in a different environment.

It was explained to the parents that there was no guarantee that a programme could help their son, and it was also emphasized that no one could foretell how far along the road to recovery he would travel. They knew, however, they had already lost this battle and that anything would be a gain to their son.

With the help of the family and volunteers and the coma-arousal nurses, a programme was commenced. He became much more awake and aware and aggressive, function was restored to both arms and legs, the tracheostomy was removed, the naso-gastric tube removed and he was fed orally. One day when one of my nurses was working with him, still in the hospice for the dying, he looked her straight in the eyes, and said, "Help me".

According to my information, he was then assessed twice with a view to be taken into a rehabilitation ward, but on both occasions the relatives were told that he was not fit for rehabilitation. It took six months to have him removed from the hospice for the dying into a nursing home, where work could be commenced on him again.

Obviously, if gains are demonstrated, there is every incentive to continue with the programme in an effort to seek further improvement.

The difficulty lies in the patient, who at the end of three months, has shown no demonstrable change. The decision-making now is variable and difficult. If the patient is a young child, it would be appropriate to continue for a further period of time. If the patient is elderly, this might not be the wisest thing to do. Who should have the final decision is a matter in which the relatives should have a major part. A book such as this cannot give you the answer, since there are so many variables.

3. The Locked-in State

The Definition of the Locked-In State

The definitive textbook on coma, *The Diagnosis of Coma and Stupor* by F. Plum and J. Posner (F.A. Davis and Co., Philadelphia, 1980), defines this condition as " . . . a state in which selective supranuclear motor deefferentation produces paralysis of all four extremities and the lower cranial nerves without interfering with consciousness. The voluntary motor paralysis prevents the subject from communicating by word or body movement."

What this means is that the motor nerves from the brain have been damaged usually in the brainstem and the muscles are paralysed preventing speech or body movement.

The difference between the locked-in state and the vegetative state is that the patient is not only awake, but also gives the impression of being aware of his environment.

The difference between a locked-in state and a spinal cord injury is that in the spinal cord injury the patient can usually speak; with the locked-in state, the patient cannot.

As its name implies, the patient is conscious (that is, *awake and aware*), but locked into a body which is virtually non-functional from a motor point of view. By this I mean that the person can receive sensation through eyes, ears, skin, muscles, etc., and can understand or comprehend a significant part of the input through the sense organs but cannot respond.

In the following diagram, the block in the cybernetic loop is shown.

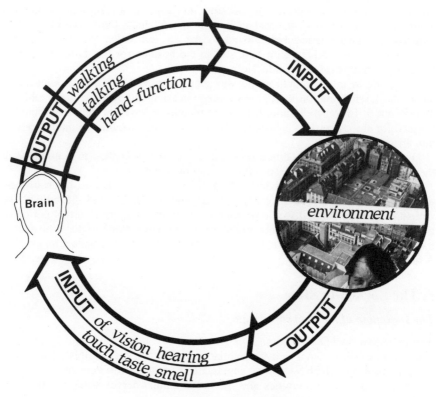

Fig. 23.2. The Locked-in State

Often it is very difficult to determine how much the patient can understand, and many of these patients are treated as though they have no ability to perceive or comprehend. Plum and Posner comment that to the unwary, this condition "can easily give the false impression of coma . . . ."

Once again it is the relatives who are more adept at the diagnosis than the professional. Because of their love and time commitments, the relatives and close friends are able to notice small changes in the patient which may be very significant. If the patient cannot talk, cannot move arms or legs, blinking to request or even moving the eyes may be the only identifiable signs of communication. There may also, of course, be some facial emotional expression which can be very important in discerning the possibility of thought and communication.

The Approaches to the Patient in the Locked-in State

The two approaches to the patient in this state are either to do nothing or to attempt to restore function. If a trial of restoration is attempted, the same type of conditions should apply as indicated in the persistent vegetative state. It is of great importance

230

to read the section How the Brain Functions, and then to chart the patient out in the Questionnaire in Chapter 9. The techniques detailed in the section The Therapy can then be used in an appropriate manner.

Conclusion

Within the health care system the diagnosis of the persistent vegetative state or locked-in state categorizes the patient as "lost", with consequent relegation to a terminal-care facility or nursing home. This solves the problem for the doctor, but not for the patient, nor the relatives, nor the community, which bears the cost of life maintenance for the remainder of the life. This often amounts to millions of dollars per patient.

In my opinion every reasonable effort must be made to improve the state of the patient, and both the patient and the family should be closely supported by all health-care professionals during this time.

SECTION G

OTHER IMPORTANT INFORMATION

CHAPTER 24

SOME ASPECTS OF THE TRADITIONAL

MANAGEMENT AND THE OUTCOME OF SEVERE

BRAIN INJURY

One reason head injuries present such a serious problem is that they are so widely dispersed through the health care system that no one person or even any one discipline sees the problem as a whole. . . . Consequently the problem tends to be left in the hope that it will be solved by someone else.

> Professor Bryan Jennett, Professor of Neurosurgery, Glasgow University, Scotland.(*Head Injuries — An Integrated Approach*, Ed.Dinning, T. Connelley, T. John Wiley and Sons, Brisbane, New York, Chichester, Toronto, 1981.)

Severe brain injury is occupying more and more medical attention in the world. As the realisation dawns that this modern-day epidemic is here to stay and that a solution must be found, the resources of governments are slowly being turned towards this hitherto neglected area. It is unlikely that as you read this book, sufficient resources will be available to help you with your problem and therefore I have consistently stated that YOU must move to deal with it.

The importance of early resuscitation

Unfortunately, rapid attention to the patient at the site of the accident and rapid transport to competent care is not necessarily the normal occurrence with severe brain injury. Often there are delays. In many countries, the problem of delayed resuscitation still remains extremely important and little attempt has been made to resolve the problem by more effective action.

There is evidence to indicate that "rapid evacuation to a neurosurgical centre, with prompt assessment by CT scanning and initiation of definitive treatment, can prevent or even reverse secondary brain injury". H.Levin, A.Benton, R.Grossman, *Neuro behavioural Consequences of Closed Head Injury*, Oxford University Press, 1982.

Quick retrieval and resuscitation is seen as a very important factor in attending to the brain-injured with a significant effect on the death rate and probably also on

233

the general outcome of the survivors. In some parts of the world, the evacuation of head-injured from the site of the accident is now carried out with the use of helicopters. Besides the rapid resuscitation "on site," the patient is in a neurosurgical hospital in less than one hour.

The effects of rapid resuscitation are threefold. It provides;

1. Rapid attention to intracranial problems.

Rapid intervention has a significant effect on the patients with intracranial bleeding from an extradural source. The bleeding here is under arterial pressure and surgical evacuation of the blood clot can be lifesaving.

2. Rapid attention to extra-cranial problems, especially respiratory (breathing) problems.

You will recall that extracranial means outside the skull.

Rapid attention to breathing difficulties is of great importance. Breathing can be affected in two major ways.

Often the airway into the brain-injured patient is blocked or partially blocked, which means that the amount of air entering the lungs is reduced. With less air going into the body, there is less oxygen going to the body organs. Some organs are very dependent upon a good supply of oxygen. The brain is particularly sensitive to oxygen lack and this reduced oxygen intake is capable of causing brain injury. This, combined with a direct hit to the brain, can be devastating.

Another way in which breathing is affected is by direct damage to the chest, either through the sternum (breast bone) or ribs. This trauma can cause lung damage, with tearing of the lung, or bleeding into the lung, or air getting between the lung and the chest wall. When there is bleeding into the lung, or blood or air getting between the lung and chest wall, the lung is compressed and the amount of lung working is reduced markedly. These events, therefore, can have very serious effects in reducing the amount of oxygen getting to the brain, thus causing brain injury, as well as being life-threatening in themselves.

3. Rapid attention to extra-cranial problems: non respiratory.

If a person has injury to an arm or leg, or especially to an internal organ such as the liver or spleen or kidney, they may lose a large amount of blood. This loss of blood brings about a fall in the blood pressure of the patient, sometimes to a dangerous level. This fall of blood pressure reduces the amount of blood, and consequently the amount of oxygen, going to the brain. This can lead to brain injury due to lack of oxygen(hypoxia = reduction in oxygen level or anoxia = no oxygen). There is also a build up of carbon dioxide in the brain which can be a disadvantage. This fall in the blood pressure also affects other vital organs such as the heart, kidneys, etc., and their ability to function is reduced so the patient goes into a state of "surgical shock" due to the loss of blood. This surgical shock can have a very severe effect on the patient who is brain-injured.

Dr B.Selecki, Visiting Neurosurgeon, Prince Henry Hospital, Sydney, Australia, summed up the position in 1979 when he said, "The present neurosurgical literature on the topic is now abundant in reports indicating that half of all deaths from head injury are associated with preventable factors such as airway obstruction, hypovolaemia (reduced amount of circulating blood leading to low blood pressure), with resulting cerebral hypoxia (lack of oxygen to the brain) and added cerebral damage in the acute stage." (B.Selecki, *Head Injuries — An Integrated Approach,* Ed.Dinning, T. Connelley, T. John Wiley and Sons, Brisbane, New York, Chichester, Toronto. 1981.)

This whole area of immediate post trauma resuscitation is obviously outside your control but it is probably worth your while to find out the facts regarding your patient. Find out the time of the accident, the delay until roadside resuscitation was commenced, how expert were the providers of that resuscitation, the method of transport to an appropriate hospital, the time involved in this stage of management, whether resuscitation was continued during this time, and whether there were any delays at the hospital. This is valuable information for you to have. If there was any unsatisfactory component of the management, you should identify it and discuss it with the appropriate authorities.

Survival and general outcome

It is important for you to know what is the likely outcome of severe brain injury if there is not a heavy input from you or your family and friends. Undoubtedly, within the statistics given in world literature there is a proportion of patients who receive stimulation from relatives and friends, often to a great extent, and I personally know people who have carried out coma arousal therapy naturally and successfully without any real input from a professional. As far as I am aware, there have been no medical studies carried out which measure the effect of having the family involved in therapy.

It is difficult to compare results from different hospital facilities since the pathology and the management of no two head injuries are the same and also because the assessing and measuring devices are too coarse to allow correct comparisons. However, even assuming the very best results are obtainable with consistency, the results are still very dismaying.

The information which you need is;

1. What are the possibilities of survival with severe brain injury?
2. What are the possibilities of a good outcome with severe brain injury?
3. Is it possible that you may be able to improve the outcome?

The following information covering the first two points is taken from a chart in the book, *Neurobehavioural Consequences of Closed Head Injury,* H. Levin, A.Benton, R.Grossman. Oxford University Press 1982.

The patients referred to in the chart in this book were all in coma for a period of more than six hours and were rated 7 or below on the Glasgow Coma Scale. This information was obtained through the setting up of an International Coma Data Bank which eventually included over 1000 patients from Glasgow in the UK, the Netherlands and Los Angeles in the USA. San Diego results, which were not associated with the International Coma Data Bank, have been included.

There has been some criticism of the criteria for admission to the study. Some neurosurgeons considered them too restrictive. Especially does this apply to the fact that even if the patient opened an eye (which is a very primitive function), the patient was excluded from the survey. Dr Donald Becker, M.D., Neurosurgeon of Richmond, Virginia, USA makes this point in the *Journal of Neurosurgery*, Vol.4, no.4,1979. as a comment to an article entitled "Prognosis of Patients with Severe Head Injury," by Jennett B., Teasdale G., Braakman R., Minderhoud J., Heiden J., and Kurze T.

Dr Becker says, "In an effort to assure that only patients with severe head injuries were included in their study, the authors limited themselves to studying only the very worst cases, which represent a relatively small percentage of patients who suffer major traumatic brain damage. Most patients in their data bank had sustained extensive irreversible brain damage."

This all points to what I have said before, that the variables can be very difficult, if not impossible, to equate. However, the results of patients in coma for six hours or over, from the various centres, were;

In Glasgow,	52%	of patients died
	2%	were vegetative
	8%	were severely disabled
	17%	were moderately disabled
	22%	made a good recovery
	101%	(?)

In The Netherlands

	52%	of patients died
	1%	were vegetative
	5%	were severely disabled
	15%	were moderately disabled
	27%	made a good recovery
	100%	

In Los Angeles

	49%	of patients died
	5%	were vegetative
	18%	were severely disabled
	14%	were moderately disabled
	14%	made a good recovery
	100%	

In San Diego

	36%	of patients died
	4%	were vegetative
	8%	were severely disabled
	10%	were moderately disabled
	42%	made a good recovery
	100%	

Information from Richmond, Virginia, a major neuroscience centre in the USA, is also available, but apparently includes some patients who were in coma for less than six hours. The results therefore are not strictly comparable, but may still be of value.

In Richmond (series 1)

30%	of patients died
2%	were vegetative
8%	were severely disabled
24%	were moderately disabled
36%	made a good recovery
100%	

In Richmond (Series 2)

34%	of patients died
3%	were vegetative
7%	were severely disabled
11%	were moderately disabled
45%	made a good recovery
100%	

Function and outcome

No one would dispute that to save a patient's life is of value. That value drops enormously if the patient remains in the vegetative state or is so severely disabled as to be "locked-in". The success must be then seen as a pyrrhic victory of which few people can be proud and with which no one can be satisfied. If new technology can provide a higher survival rate, the medical profession, the government and the community are obliged to seek the best outcome for the survivors. This makes sense not only from the human point of view but also from the financial point of view. Severely brain-injured patients are an enormous cost to the community financially. Insurance payments for some patients in certain countries are well into the millions of dollars per patient. Even if this lump sum payment is not made, the cost of care for the brain-injured person who survives for decades is in the millions of dollars per patient. It is economic commonsense to strive for the best outcome.

That this commonsense is not present in most countries has been implied by Professor Bryan Jennett of the University of Glasgow who writes, "Although head injury is 10 times more frequent than spinal injuries, there is much less chance that the victims of head injury will be fortunate enough to find a coherent and expertly conceived rehabilitation programme." (Rosenthal, M., Griffiths, R. Bond, M. Miller J.D. *Rehabilitation of the Head Injured Adult*, F.A.Davis Company, 1983.)

One of the most important research papers on the outcome of severe brain injury is that of Professor Jennett, Dr Snoek, Professor Bond and Dr Brooks who reported their findings on the outcome of 150 *survivors* of severe brain injury in an article entitled "Disability after Severe Head Injury:Observations on the use of the Glasgow Outcome Scale." *Journal of Neurology, Neurosurgery, and Psychiatry*, 44, 285-293, 1981.

They write, "Some deficit was detected, albeit sometimes mild, in 97 of these 150 patients. Two thirds had personality change which in almost 30 was the only deficit.

"Disorders of verbal intellect were found to be relatively infrequent, while disorders of learning and memory, and of performance intelligence were found to be severe and persistent; these findings are in accord with several psychological studies of severe head injury."

Conclusion

In 1977, the group from The Division of Neurological Surgery, Medical College of Virginia, Virginia Commonwealth University, Richmond, Virginia, wrote in an article entitled "The Outcome from Severe Head Injury with Early Diagnosis and Intensive Management":

"The management of patients with severe head injury continues to present neurosurgeons with a major challenge; mortality and morbidity are appallingly high, and detailed neurological and psychosocial studies reveal that many apparent recoveries are in fact social tragedies." Becker, D. Miller, J. Ward, J. Greenberg, R. Young, H. Sakalas, R. *Journal of Neurosurgery* 47: 491-502,1977.

The active involvement of relatives and friends may alter these results in three ways.

1.   It is possible that if the patient can be aroused from coma more quickly, the depth and duration of the intense sensory deprivation will be lessened, with an amelioration of the devastating effects of coma.

2.   It is possible that the security of the relatives' presence during the "Fragile Period" of coma may wrap the patient in a protective cocoon, preventing or reducing the gross personality changes that seem to occur from severe brain injury.

3.   It is possible that learning and memory can be stimulated by the relatives much earlier than is presently being done and that the continuity provided by the relatives will be of great importance in obtaining better cognitive function.

This information is provided as a guide only. By this time you will be aware that although Medicine has a strong scientific component, there are large areas which are not black and white, but which are fuzzy grey. The outcome of severe brain injury is an enormous grey area. If you, and your family, and friends, can help to shift your patient out of the grey unknown, into the known, you will have done him or her an enormous loving service.

CHAPTER 25

HOW DOES THE PATIENT FEEL?

PUT ME IN YOUR HUMAN EYE

COME TASTE

THE BITTER TEARS

THAT I CRY

TOUCH ME

WITH YOUR HUMAN HAND

HEAR ME WITH YOUR EAR

BUT NOTICE ME

DAMN YOU

NOTICE ME I'M HERE

ric masten
(*Looking Out / Looking In,
Interpersonal Communication,*
Adler, R. Towne, N. Holt,
Rinehart and Winston, 1975)

John was moribund in coma for six weeks following a severe infection of the brain known as encephalitis. He was not expected to live and when it became obvious that he was going to survive, the medical opinion was that he would be vegetative. He has provided the information on how it feels from the inside of coma and the awakening period. Intertwined with John's story is that of Yvonne, his wife.

John says, "I am often asked what is it like to be in coma? I truly have no recollections of that period, but I do have recollections, some vivid and some vague, of the period of awakening and the period following the awakening."

The diagnosis of encephalitis, given to Yvonne, was followed by the doctor's prognosis given in as comforting a manner as possible, that "John cannot live till morning."

Yvonne had considerable support from her parents and very special friends, some of whom were in the nursing profession.

John remained in a critical condition for weeks and it was during this time, while John was still attached to the life support equipment in the intensive care ward, that

Yvonne encountered those hopeless words from a doctor, "All this is a waste of time."

After four weeks in the intensive care unit, it was suggested to Yvonne that the experimental research going on into Coma Arousal, might be worth trying. I well recall the first meeting with Yvonne. I had been to the ward to have a preliminary look at John and was just leaving the room when she came to the door. I had been told a little about her by the attending physician who had expressed his admiration. It was impressed on me that she was a woman with an enormous love for her husband and also a person with exceptional self control. After meeting her I agreed with his judgment.

It was carefully explained to Yvonne that there was no promise of success but that there was a chance to wake John up if he was indeed "in there."

John says, "Indeed I was, and although I have no recollection of the coma arousal techniques, even though I am now familiar with them, it was around this time that I started to have dreams and what would have appeared to be hallucinations to those observing me."

Let John now tell some pertinent parts of his story.

"Why do I believe that Coma Arousal was of help to me when in coma and the period of awakening?

Having spent six weeks in coma with no sign of awakening, and having had clinical indicators of severe brain damage, beyond any hope of redemption, I am here writing to you.

Not that I attribute my life to the Coma Arousal Therapy. My life was preserved by the techniques used in the intensive care unit at Westmead Hospital. But it was during the period of awakening that Coma Arousal saved, in the least, my sanity, preserved my will to live, and brought the realisation to me that I was not forever ensconced in hell on earth.

If Florence Nightingale came back now and could see the advances in nursing due to her efforts and determination, she would be justifiably proud, that is, until she happened upon the ward full of "vegies". She would, I believe, cry. For this ward, and its lack of care, would remind her of the first ward she encountered.

In this day and age! Dirty beds? Dirty patients? Offhand attitudes by most of the medical fraternity and unfortunately some of the nurses. Not just to me and my family but to other unfortunate patients in a similar position to me.

Not all staff were understanding. Some of the things said in front of me hurt. Some of the things said to me hurt as well. I hope that they will learn that a brain injury does not kill feelings.

I know that even in the very early stages of my erratic recovery I was JOHN. I was still capable of thought, worries and cares. I needed to see my wife, for her to be close to me. I needed to see my family and friends to offset the nightmare which happened only too frequently. Not that all strangers proved unfriendly. No, but too many did.

My outrage at my treatment is not a blanket condemnation of all those involved in the care of the comatose patient. It is a condemnation of those who are too blind to see, or unwilling to see for reasons beyond my comprehension, any little sign that the patient is improving, or wants to improve.

I could see, could hear, but blurred and muffled my confused and worried brain would draw wrong conclusions from the facts presented to it.

During this awakening period I endured numerous, stupid, and to my mind, needless nightmares.

What a headache, what a hangover. I tried but could not bring my brain to focus on anything. All I could think of was that I had definitely had one too many, or a cellar too many, last night.

"Do you know the time? Do you know the date? Where are you?" Who the blazes cares, and if this fellow kneeling by the bed asking these inane questions did not know the answers to these inane questions, why in the name of all that's holy is he asking me.

I was aware one day of a well built lady working on my limbs as though I was incidental to the proceedings and saying to another, "We're only doing this 'cause She's (presumably Yvonne) a friend of Hers." Who "Her" was I had no idea at the time. I wish I could meet her to give her my thanks.

Tired of waking to a wet bed in the early hours of the morning, and discovering that the answer to my yells for help were answered by the closing of the door of my room, I asked for the catheter to be replaced. This was refused on the grounds that "I should consider myself lucky to be alive," and that "Nothing further could be done for me," and that "I would spend the rest of my life in the state I was now in." Then, "We cannot understand how you have survived this far, you are a very lucky man."

Lucky, lucky, laying here as incontinent as an old man. No. Think. Think. Make yourself think what to do. You cannot walk so jumping out the window isn't the way.

I nearly gave up. I did not give up. I could not move my body properly and certainly not in a co-ordinated fashion. My mental abilities were certainly limited. Also I was not allowed to give up. My wife and family and friends would not let me give up. I knew I could not give up.

At one stage I was advised to accept the fact that my brain was so damaged that I would never talk again. Two weeks later, I was able to ask that same person when I would be able to walk again. He said, "John, you do not understand. You will never walk. The brain damage is far too severe."

I made myself a promise. One which I would tell nobody about until I had achieved it. I was going to walk out of this hospital unaided by walking stick or crutches and definitely not in a wheelchair.

Some weeks later I walked past the person who had said that I would never talk, or walk, in the corridor. He refused to speak to me and hasn't since. I must have upset him in some way

The factors which played the greatest element in my recovery were, I believe, the intense and continued input of love and positive calming actions provided by my wife and her family and friends to my demented ravings. This input came from those I knew and could trust.

I was not driven to recovery. I was led as a horse to water that wanted only too willingly to drink but did not know how to. The thirst was as unbearable as the lack of ability and the knowledge of how to drink.

I was constantly being told that my ability to retain information was dismal. I know I was not supposed to be able to remember anything, but there was nothing in the room to read and memorise. They gave me nothing to practice on.

What an absolute pleasure it was to win something for the first time. I was tired of being treated like a second class citizen. I was able to correct one of the nurses about my medication and give my medical record number. "Aren't you a clever little boy, knowing your MRN," I was told. I was infuriated.

When I first attempted to get out of bed in an effort to walk, I was sprung by the charge sister. To say that I was given the dressing down of my life would be about right. But, this sister spoke to me as though I was an adult. A normal sane responsible adult. This was the first time someone had spoken to me in that way. I cried.

To mention the many aspects of negative attitudes given by people to me, both in and out of the hospital environment would be tedious and repetitious. One of the curious things was that as I progressed, the less many of my previous caregivers wanted to know me. It was as if my survival and consequent failure to follow their predictions of the vegetative state had confounded them.

The second question I am often asked is, "Do you think Coma Arousal works?"

I don't know. What I do know from my own experience is that the period of awakening from coma is traumatic, frightening and regretfully not understood by many of the hospital staff. Statements made by relatives and a couple of patients to me reinforce this view. It is a time when the known has to be brought to the patient's attention, when support in the early stages of awakening and recovery are so important, when a person will respond far better to a known face, voice, touch, and when a stranger's presence will evoke fear and the desire to run, but you cannot.

Difficult at times, I agree that I was. At times my expectations of my capabilities were far in excess of my physical and mental abilities. I am sure that it was from the input around me, from family, friends and the Coma Arousal team that I realised that the question of improvement was limited mainly by my attitude and not just the limitations apparently placed on me by the insult to my brain and the ensuing wastage of muscle.

Yes, I believe Coma Arousal was of great benefit to me."

CHAPTER 26

HOW DO THE RELATIVES COPE?

Therefore, strengthen your feeble arms and weak knees!
Make level paths for your feet,
so that the lame may not be disabled,
but rather healed.

(Letter to the Hebrews, Chapter 12.)

There is no doubt that your lifestyle will change. No one can go through the experience of severe brain injury, neither patient nor relative, without a massive change and rearrangement of lifestyle. How you handle that change will have a very significant influence on the remainder of your life.

There are many books on the market about coping with severe stress. These are written by experts, and it is obviously valuable if you obtain one with which you feel comfortable, and use it as a constant source of reference. Here I wish to present what I have seen in this work with the brain-injured from my own experience.

Whenever there is a problem, it is a reasonable approach to weigh up the size and extent of the problem and the size and extent of the resources available to deal with the problem. No coach of a football team or a basketball team goes into a match without carefully assessing the extent and depth of the opposition and the strength of their own team. They then work out a strategy based both on the reality as they see it and the hope of what the outcome will be. So basic to both the football coach and to you are two important and dominating factors: Reality and Hope.

Reality

I have constantly brought to your attention the importance of assessing the reality of the situation. Unless you are in touch with reality, your effectiveness in helping to recover the person you love will be greatly diminished.

There are two essential realities with which you must deal. The first relates to factors concerning the PATIENT, and the second relates to factors concerning YOU.

The Reality of the Patient

Much of this book is involved in providing you with the tools for gaining information about the patient, about their condition, diagnosis, prognosis, etc., which allows you to assess the real state of the patient. Of importance also is the gaining of information which will allow you to assess the attitude and care of the physicians, nursing staff, paramedics, etc.

This information and assessment is "cold-brain" food, and you know by now that if you have cold brain functioning, your problem-solving abilities will be better than if your "hot brain" dominates.

Much of the book is also concerned with satisfying the needs of the patient. The very basis of the needs of the patient can be stated from Dr William Glasser's book, *Reality Therapy* (Perennial Library, Harper and Row, New York, London, 1975), "At all times in our lives we must have at least one person who cares about us and whom we care for ourselves."

Reality for You

Every person has

Mental
Physical
Social and
Spiritual resources.

These resources can be weakened or strengthened, depending upon the desires of that person. These resources are dynamic and constantly changing and need to be in balance with each other.

Mental Resources

Mental resources are both intellectual and emotional. Your cold brain and your hot brain functions. They work together. There is no doubt that what happens in the intellectual or thinking part of your brain affects the emotional part of your brain in a tremendous way. There is no doubt that the emotional or feeling part of your brain affects the intellectual part of your brain in a tremendous way. How you feel is a reflection of how you think. How you feel also determines how you think. If you want to feel good, you must think of how good you feel. This is known as "Self-talk". Dr Albert Ellis and Dr Robert Harper have in their book, *A New Guide to Rational Living* (Prentice Hall International, Inc., London, 1975), a chapter entitled, "You Feel the Way You Think". It is worthwhile reading.

Self-talk

In other chapters I have stressed the importance of the various "personal space zones", and how vital they are to us and how aware we must be when we transgress into the personal bubble of the patient. There is another space zone which we have not delved into. It is called "Inner Space". It is inside your own mind. Your thoughts and feelings are in inner space. Only one person can let anyone intrude into your inner space and that is you.

You can either self-talk yourself into feeling good or feeling bad. You can self-talk yourself into feeling unhappy or happy. You can self-talk yourself into being productive or unproductive. You can self-talk yourself into being effective or ineffective. You can self-talk yourself into trying or not trying. You can self-talk yourself into success or failure. You can self-talk yourself into stopping or going. You can self-talk yourself into action or apathy. You can self-talk yourself into winning or losing. The choice belongs to one person — YOU.

Do not forget:

YOU WIN OR LOSE BY THE WAY YOU CHOOSE.

If you choose to venture into this minefield of severe brain injury, you must do so with determination.

If you choose to venture into this minefield of severe brain injury, you must do so with courage.

If you choose to venture into this minefield of severe brain injury, you must do so with endurance.

Who decides whether you have determination, courage or endurance? You do. No one else can decide for you. The choice is yours.

Therefore, thoughts which are not positive about yourself and your capabilities should be eradicated from your mind as soon as they occur. You may need to make up some positive affirmations which you repeat to yourself routinely every day, and some which you repeat at times of stress. You may not be able to control what other people say about you, but you can surely control what you say about yourself.

Other People's Talk

You know that the world is constantly trying to "put you down". The world is constantly trying to place people into either winner or loser categories. Any person who has a relative who is severely brain-injured is seen as a loser. How else could you or your family be seen? You suddenly are viewed as having an albatross around your neck, like the Ancient Mariner.

So you must listen to what is being said, monitor it, sort out the gold from the dross. Pick up the gold and discard the dross. If you are unsure of what is being said to you, or unsure about a person's attitude, ask for clarification. You are about important business, you need to be as clear in your mind as possible on all important points. If you feel that you are not receiving correct information, ask for information from another source. If you feel that you are not being listened to, ask to be listened to. I well remember having an interview with a Senator whom I felt was not paying attention to what I was saying. I said to him, "You are not listening to what I am saying." He replied, "Yes I am, I was just wondering if this is not similar to the story of Ignatz Semmelweiss." He certainly listened from that point on.

If you have paid attention to other people's talk, have found the talk to be incorrect, especially if it is antagonistic to you personally, recall those words of John Rogers which dispense with other people's opinions,

WHAT YOU SAY ABOUT ME IS NONE OF *MY* BUSINESS.

You are who you are: a unique individual who has entered an unknown world. You possess all the faults and attributes of your humanness and your uniqueness. You are of great value and worth. You must not be destroyed by the opinions of other people.

Visualization

We are all familiar with the saying, "The thought is mother to the action." Perhaps it is more accurate to say, "The thought is mother to the visualization, which is mother to the action."

Creative visualization may help you immensely. There are many books written upon this subject, most of which are easily available. Shakti Gawain in *Creative Visualization* (Bantam Books, 1979) writes that *"Creative visualization* is the technique of using your imagination to create what you want in your life."

This method of channelling your thinking into pictures has been known for centuries. So much of our thought and language is easily changed to pictures. You can use creative visualization from the moment you awake in the morning until the moment you go to sleep. Commence on waking and visualize in your mind what are likely to be the happenings of the day. If there is something of great significance, see yourself in your imagination actually heading to the place, see yourself walking in the door, see yourself talking to the people, discussing what is going to occur, exploring the possibilities and solutions. Your mind, once it commences to run with this process of imagination, will let you have a "dry run" before the actual events take place. You can also "dry-run" as much and as many times as you like. You can also vary the methods which you use in dealing with the problems in your mind's eye.

Some people find it easier to think of a television set in their head, on which they see the pictures actually unfolding. If this works for you, do it.

It is also often worth-while at the end of the day to reverse the procedure and go through, in your brain, all the important things which happened and identify the areas of special concern. You have already been asked to do this by using your diary. Another way is to talk over each day's happenings with some close relative or friend.

There are some people who believe that creative visualization can help in another way. I am not sure about what they propose, but I would comment that no harm is likely to come from it. These people propose that your thoughts also influence the person whom you are thinking about. Therefore, they maintain that it is worth while visualizing the patient getting better and doing this each day. My only counsel here would be that you should stay in touch with reality and visualize the restoring process slowly and not miraculously. However, I may be wrong, due to my own limitations on visualization and its possibilities.

It is possible also that the patient out of coma, but with gross limitations of function, may be able to creatively visualize himself or herself and improve function. Many top athletes now use the technique of visualizing to enhance their performance, and the same principles should apply to any person, athletic or not. A book which is worth checking out is *The Inner Game of Tennis* by W. Timothy Gallway (Bantam Press, 1974).

Meditation

There are a myriad of techniques on meditation. By entering into the subconscious mind, many people claim to be able to rid themselves of their anxieties and stress and worries, and enter back into the external world refreshed. This may be the thing for you.

The Importance of Forgiveness

Forgiveness is so often presented to us as being among the most difficult things in the world to accomplish. It is through forgiveness that we open the door to strength. When you have been hurt, the more you harbour that hurt, the more it eats into you. If you have hurt yourself, you harbour guilt. If you have been hurt by others, you harbour resentment. Both are destructive. Every person who has a brain-injured relative has reason to feel guilty. We all start the process of "If only I had not . . . this would not have happened." We commence the process in relation to events immediately preceding the accident, and we follow them further back through the years, even to times when the patient was a young child. We question why we did not see the significance of a previous event, why we did not take notice when something happened, why we did not spend more time with the person. Unless we have obviously done something which directly and through intent was designed to harm the patient, we must forgive ourselves. Sometimes we need spiritual guidance to do this, but do it we must, otherwise guilt and resentment will weaken us.

Other people we must forgive are those who in some way were concerned with the lifestyle of the patient before the accident, even those directly involved in the tragic events. It is important to work on this whole matter. Frequently we need to self-talk our way into forgiveness of other people. We may even need to visualize the coming-together of the person who has caused the hurt and ourselves.

The Importance of the "Now"

It has been said, "The past is over, the future is to come, we only have the NOW." This very precious moment of this instant, this minute, this hour, this day. No one would dispute the importance of the past, for it sets our lines of direction for the present and the future: it is our history. No one disputes the importance of the future, nor the importance of planning in a sensible way for that future. But it is the present NOW in which we live. Time spent looking backwards can be valuable, for we learn so much. Time spent looking forward is essential, otherwise we drift like a rudderless ship. But we are only living in the present, the here and now. This time has been called "The Precious Moment", and it should not be wasted. It can never be replaced. So, while you must look back and look forward, attempt in every way to live in the present, because that is where the changing reality remains. It is also the only time in which you can act and accomplish the things you need to do.

Be aware of the old saying, "My job is not to look dimly in the distance, but to do what lies clearly at hand."

In a practical sense this means that while your life has been markedly altered by the brain injury, you must maintain as much of your old familiar way of life as possible and, indeed, look to learn or do something new. One lady I respect a great deal has coped with the fact of her son's severe brain injury by breeding and showing dogs. Others take up painting or music or meditation. Others maintain themselves in a part-time job. Others go back to their studies and do further courses.

During the early stages after the brain injury it is most unlikely that you will either feel like doing any of the above or have the time to do so. But do not separate yourself from the life which you know and which you must still develop.

There will be times when you just want to sit and think and feel the anguish and the agony of what has happened. No one could deny you time to do this, to go through your feelings and explore them. But do not get lost in them. Do not suffocate in them for long periods. While it is important to look inwards and to bring out the grief and the hurt, do not stay imprisoned in your feelings, for it will help neither the patient nor you. If you are becoming bound in, seek some help from friends or from understanding professional people.

Physical Wellbeing

Your own physical wellbeing is of paramount importance. This means that you must look after yourself, so that you are able to participate in looking after the person you love. Exercise is of great importance. We are physical animals, and our bodies need to be worked and not to soften. Keep up any exercise programme you have going, and if you do not exercise, then start to do so. Walking is very worth while, and can become a ritual if you walk at the same time each day along a chosen path.

Your diet is also important. You should have regular meals as much as possible, and since you are under stress you may need to have some additional vitamins. You should consult an expert on this matter.

Adequate sleep is essential. There are natural substances which can help you sleep, but there are times when you may need to resort, for a limited period, to sleeping pills. The more you can do without these the better as most do become addictive. Many people find that relaxation exercises and meditation before going to bed are of value.

Social Wellbeing

Social interaction should be actively sought. There is a great temptation to withdraw from social contact and become buried in the problems which you face. This is natural and, at times, necessary. Social contact is important, however. Do not forget also that friends and acquaintances are often unsure how to approach you and will tend not to want to disturb you and may stay away. Do not be concerned about this, but make contact with them. Ask them to do something to help you. Draw them into what you are doing, if they are willing to help. Many people will not be able to help for reasons which are quite legitimate. Respect their feelings. Recognize always that people are able to lift you from your problem into new thoughts and actions.

Spiritual Growth

We are brought up in a scientifically oriented world. The spiritual often does not get a "look in". This does not mean it is not there. Just because we do not recognize something does not mean that it does not exist. I have been brought up in the Christian tradition, and my knowledge of other spiritual lives and works is almost non-existent. This does not mean that I would not recognize the value in them. I am sure that many of the world's religions have much in common and can be a source of great help and guidance to people. If you are in tune with a spiritual presence, you may gain great benefit.

You may never have had anything to do with the spiritual aspects of life. In this case you must tread warily. If the "fruit of the Spirit is love, joy, peace, patience, kindness, goodness, faithfulness, gentleness and self-control" (The Letter to the Galatians, Chapter 5, v. 22-23), these are the fruits you should look for in any spiritual exercise. The three great spiritual qualities that Paul also writes about, in his first Letter to the Corinthians, Chapter 13, are Faith, Hope and Love.

Faith

Faith may be the most intimate thing in our life. Belief in a Power greater than human power plays an enormous part in the lives of many people. The link between Humankind and God is prayer, in whatever form this may take. It may be public prayer or private prayer. It may be a yearning to be in touch with the Power of the Universe. Faith is a unique and personal quality for each person, and I am not able to venture into your faith. I do know, however, many people whose faith in God and in God's purpose for their life, and the life of the person who is brain-injured, has been of the very greatest importance in recovery. This is something which you must explore yourself, and I would not wish to intrude on it.

Hope

Hope has already been dealt with to a certain extent in an early chapter. It is so important that it merits further attention. It is a truism to say, "Without hope the people perish."

Emile Brunner has written:

What oxygen is for the lungs,
such is hope for the meaning of human life.
Take oxygen away
and death occurs through suffocation;
take hope away
and humanity is constricted through lack of breath;
despair comes in,
spelling the paralysis of intellectual and spiritual powers
by a feeling of the senselessness
and purposelessness of existence.
As the fate of the human organism

is dependent on the supply of oxygen,
so the fate of humanity
is dependent upon its supply of hope.

Dr Arnold Hutschnecker, M.D., in his book on *Hope* (G.P. Putnam's Sons, New York, 1981) writes of two types of Hope: passive hope and active hope.

Passive hope is the daydreaming, unreal hope which people hold when they are not in touch with reality. They wish that something would happen, but take no active steps to bring the wish about. They are dependent upon others achieving, without having any significant input themselves. Dr Hutschnecker writes, "Passive hope is the bread and wine of the poor. It is the beautiful fantasy world of children, of the oppressed, the fearful . . . While people with active hope use their strength and imagination to make their dreams come true, people with passive hope watch with admiration the pioneers building cities and bridges and hospitals and kindergartens, while they never dare to spread their wings."

Active hope is a mobilization of resources both internal and external, a recognition of reality with all its problems, a determination to engage in the conflict, the patience and endurance to pursue the objectives, the recognition that victory does not always go to the brave, but always to have the hunger to strive to succeed.

Every reasonable avenue which can be explored should be entered, every bit of strength and knowledge should be sought, every support mechanism should be used to activate hope in yourself, the patient, relatives and friends.

Love

Amongst the most beautiful of the world's literature is the Letter to the Corinthians, (1st Corinthians, Chapter 13). I can add no further to the following;
"Love is patient,
love is kind.
It does not envy,
it is not proud.
It is not rude,
it is not self seeking,
it is not easily angered,
it keeps no record of wrongs.
Love does not delight in evil
but rejoices with the truth.
It always protects,
always trusts,
always hopes,
always perseveres,
And now these three remain:
faith, hope and love.
But the greatest of these is
love."

Failure

Can there be failure? There will always be some patients who do not respond. It is as yet unknown whether this is due to the injury being so severe that nothing can be done, or whether it is due to our failure to be able to provide what is needed due to lack of knowledge or lack of facilities. Some patients will remain in coma in the persistent vegetative state or will be so severely brain-injured and "locked-in" that they are unable to communicate.

One of the comforting thoughts which help some people is the knowledge that they have done everything they possibly can in an attempt to arouse the patient and restore function. Some may see this as of no importance but I am convinced that the fact that a determined effort has been made is helpful in reducing the guilt that comes so easily but which is so uncalled for in the relatives.

Coping with such a horrendous predicament as the vegetative state must be amongst the most difficult things which any person can be asked to do. You have to ask yourself which way to take. You have a choice of two roads to follow — you can either choose to survive or you can choose to die mentally, physically, emotionally, socially, spiritually. To withdraw from life, to wither away. It is your right to do this if you consider it is the way for you.

Before you choose to withdraw, you are committed to seeing what are the benefits of your withdrawal to the patient, to your husband/wife/children. Will your removal from the scene be of help to them and in what way? You need to discuss this with them individually and collectively. You need to explore deeply because the question of your involvement is of such immense importance to so many people.

In their book, *How Can I Help?*, Ram Dass and Paul Gorman (Rider and Company, Great Britain, 1986) ask this very question.

"And, finally, what of those moments when we question whether we've anything useful for others? What do we really have to offer, what do we really have to give? Everything, it turns out. Everything. If within each of us is that essence of Being which is in all things — call it God, Life, Energy, Consciousness — so we have to share it with one another.

"It could mean that . . . they can feel in who we are the reassurance that they are not simply isolated entities, separate selves, lonely beings, cut off from everything and everyone else. They can feel us in there with them. They can feel the comfort that we are all of us in this together. They have the chance to know in moments of great pain that nevertheless we are Not Separate.

"When all else fails, when we've done what we can, we still have this essential reassurance to offer one another."

If you choose, there is the possibility of your growing in awareness of life and of being a resource for other people in need. It is possible to take the hurt which is within you and to transform the whole of your life by changing it from a negative to a positive force. To do this requires an intent to constantly seek the good in every situation, to develop that good, leaving all the bad. It is really seeking a situation where everybody wins. We come back to the concept once again of the Wounded Healer.

Conclusion

Is it all worth it? No one can answer that question for you. It is your privilege to make the choice.

YOU ARE A PERSON OF VALUE AND WORTH

Do not abdicate the choice to anyone else. Listen to what people tell you. Listen to your own heart for it will tell you the truth. Logic should not be the dominant thought in these unusual circumstances. No one can allocate numbers to the mass of different factors which would need to be taken into consideration to make a logical decision. It is what YOU want to do which is important. It is how you feel about the whole proposition which should determine your choice. If you choose not to stay involved with your severely brain-injured patient, no one can force you to and no one should attempt to do so. If you wish to remain heavily involved with your brain-injured relative, that is your choice and no one should attempt to move you from your position. In either choice, it is quite possible that you may not cope for periods of quite long duration. This is normal. As has been said, "It is insane to stay sane in an insane situation. You have to work through the insanity of the situation. No one else can do it for you. You may need help. Seek it out and use it, but you be the judge of what you need and what you want. If you need to be transformed to deal with this problem seek out a reputable transformation group or a Centre for Attitudinal Healing. This may be your way of growing and stretching in your total being, and it may be the way in which you can help the other people that you love.

CHAPTER 27

WHAT MAY BEAT YOU IN THE SYSTEM AND HOW

TO DEAL WITH IT

Problems are what you see
when you take your eye
off the objective.

The Background to the Medical System

The medical profession consists of people who are highly trained, highly motivated and highly concerned about their patients. There are always exceptions to the rule, but the majority of physicians and surgeons are competent and caring.

Like everyone else, those in the medical profession wish to succeed in their work and it is largely because of their skill and dedication that there are many people today who owe their lives to the great advances in modern Medicine. The advent of antibiotics, anaesthetics, blood transfusion, organ transplants, in vitro fertilisation, are all testimony to the power of medical science and technology.

While no one would wish to detract from these dramatic advances, these achievements have directed the attention of both the public and the professions on to science as the great cure-all of the world's problems. Consequently, modern medical schools and universities are producing physicians more inclined to see the patient as a physiological mechanism which has gone wrong, than as a person who needs help. This bias to the scientific method has produced a race of physicians whose first question is always "What scientific evidence is there for this statement?" or "How can this be proven?"

These questions are acceptable as part of life, but life consists of more than science. Life consists of human relationships. Of love, peace, patience, joy, tolerance, forbearing, etc., as St Paul has identified in his Letter to the Galatians. Can these things be measured scientifically? I think not. They are dynamics which are beyond scientific measure and yet they are the most important aspects of life.

Much medicine practised, even in the highly technological hospitals at the forefront of scientific endeavour, is also non scientific.

The Severely Brain-Injured and the System

With the patient in coma, or severely brain-injured and disabled, the very best of medical resources have been expended, but the end result is frequently not seen as successful, either by the relatives or the physician. Because the profession is not yet aware that the problem which must now be treated is a new one, it continues to treat the old. This has been dealt with in the Chapter 4. The profession treats the Internal Affairs Department of the patient admirably, but is still not aware that it is the External Affairs Department of the patient which is in a state of failure.

Your difficulty is that, firstly, the physician attending to your patient may not even be aware that she/he has a new problem to treat and secondly that even if she/he becomes aware, she/he will be unlikely to know what to do about it productively.

Not only is it that your physician does not know, it is very likely that the nursing staff and paramedical departments also do not know. Neither do the administrators of the hospital.

In the final analysis, the administrators of the system of health care, when the utmost has been provided for the patient, as they see it, must weigh up the cost/benefit of keeping the patient in hospital. If there is no obvious benefit to the patient to be gained by acute hospitalisation, they are committed to removing the patient from the acute hospital system into a long term care system, that is hospice, terminal care or nursing home.

The most convenient way for you to look at the potential problems in the system, which you will need to deal with are to identify problems with TIME, PLACE, and PERSON.

TIME

There are four critical time periods which you must consider. These are;

A. The length of time the patient is in coma

I have stressed repeatedly that the longer the patient remains in coma, the worse appears to be the outcome. Therefore, it is imperative that you should talk to the attending doctor as soon as possible so you may commence work with the patient. "Do not fiddle and hope", (as the placards on cardiac arrest say). Fiddling and hoping are not happy bedfellows. Active hope demands action. If, in your discussions with the doctor, you are constantly being told that you must wait and see what happens and that nothing else can be done, unless there are strong contraindications, you must start to take the initiative. There may be a so-called "Critical Period" after the brain injury which is when the best results can be obtained. Do not let this important time slip by without realizing it. This is discussed in Chapter 17, The Reorganisation of the Brain.

Before you take the initiative, however, it is important to be sure that the patient is out of the life-threatened condition. Your plan of action must be;

1. Within the first week, have a discussion with the doctor about the condition of the patient to determine how life-threatened he or she is.

2. If the patient is not life-threatened, ask when you can commence an arousal programme.

3. Prepare a document setting out your findings on the patient from the questionnaire, and also the proposed programme, and ask if the doctor would be

254

agreeable to your commencing a programme slowly. Indicate that you would be prepared to provide a continuing report of what you see.

4.   Maintain contact with your doctor as much as possible. If you detect any change at all in the patient, either notify him or her verbally or leave a note with the ward sister. Always keep a copy of your notes and on these show the time and date that you provided the note and to whom it was given.

B. The amount of time which can be given to the patient in an effort to arouse from coma and restore function

Once again we come back to the factors of quantity and quality of time. Effective work means both a sufficient amount and a good standard of input. While there are times when it is correct just to sit by the patient and hold his/her hand, this constitutes reassurance, not work. The only way to be sure of doing the work is to set up a programme which is realistic and effective and to stick to it as much as possible. There are always times when the patient cannot receive therapy due to other hospital requirements. Respect these times, but do all in your power to ensure that the work gets done.

C. The length of time the patient is kept in the acute hospital

Often what happens is that the patient is left in the acute hospital because there is nowhere else to go or because no one considers some more active input is necessary. It is your business to be aware of these potential problems. Some comatose patients are kept in the acute hospitals for 3 — 6 months as a routine purely to establish the diagnosis of the persistent vegetative state before being shipped off to terminal care or nursing home facilities. You must not let this happen to your patient. You must know what is proposed at all times.

D. The time when the patient reaches a "plateau"

You will often hear the physician say that a patient is making no more progress and has reached a "plateau". This implies that the patient has come to the limit of his or her ability and that it is unlikely that there will be any further improvement in function. It is my impression that the first thing to consider when this condition of plateauing occurs, is the programme of work being done with the patient. Often the reason patients fail to make further improvement is that they are bored and have lost motivation. This is the time for that new look and a changed approach.

Linked in with the above is the so-called end point of improvement. Some extremely important work has been done in brain injury by the team from Glasgow of Professor Bryan Jennett, Professor of Neurosurgery, Professor Graham Teasdale, Professor Michael Bond and Dr Neil Brooks. In many ways, they have put severe brain injury on to the medical map. In 1981, in *The Journal of Neurology, Neurosurgery, and Psychiatry* (Vol 44. p. 285-293), they reported their findings on a group of 1000 brain-injured patients. The title was "Disability after Severe Head Injury: Observations on the Use of the Glasgow Outcome Scale". Briefly, they found that patients improved mainly in the first six months after injury and that there appeared to be little improvement after this time. The influence of these physicians was so great that this medical article became an edict which is still quoted today very widely, so it is possible that your own doctor will quote these facts at you. The most important thing to consider, however, is, what was the after care treatment of these patients, for you should by now be well aware that the environment in which the brain-injured patient is placed is critical in determining the outcome. Undoubtedly, these patients were provided with the best in neurosurgical care during the acute stage but the quality of their post acute care may have been extremely variable. (The facts relating to this are not discussed in the article.)

PLACE

There are several factors here. Place can mean all aspects from the position of the patient in bed through to the transfer and placement in another hospital. Remember, the patient is not in the position of being able to make a request as to where he/she would like to be, or in what position. You have to be sensitive to the needs of the patient. Do not forget how vulnerable the patient is.

Hospital Bed

No one likes to be kept stationary or fixed in position. Make sure that the patient is moved around in the bed and also sat up. Also he or she should be taken out of bed and placed in a chair for substantial periods of the morning and afternoon. Do your utmost to get the patient out of bed, even if you have to request some help from the nursing staff to physically make the move.

Hospital Room

The room for the patient can also become a prison. Being put into a wheel-chair and taken out of the room is a liberating action. Recognise that there may be some antagonism to the patient being taken out to the lifts or even outside into the sun and the fresh air. Speak to the ward sister and seek her co-operation. If the patient has an infection there may only be certain parts of the hospital to which he/she may go. Always enquire first about the areas which may not be safe. Often you will find that,if the patient has a tracheostomy, the hospital will want to ensure that a sucker and oxygen is available and also that a nurse is present at all times. This is reasonable and you should co-operate as much as possible.There may be legal as well as medical factors which dictate this requirement. If the hospital is unable to provide you with a nurse, you may be able to make private arrangements.

Hospital

I have stressed that acute hospitals are not the ideal place in which a brain-injured patient can recover once out of the life-threatened state. Such a patient, not to mention the relatives, is a difficulty to all concerned after they have been an inpatient for a period of weeks. Especially is this so if there appears to be no improvement or little improvement in their condition. Of course, if the patient remains life-threatened then the acute hospital remains the appropriate institution, but not otherwise. Therefore, as soon as you possibly can, you should begin to seek alternative care and accommodation. This does not mean that you should take the responsibility of moving the patient unless circumstances are very difficult. This is the responsibility of the medical profession. You should however, be aware of what is, and is not, available.

PEOPLE

Concerned people are your greatest strength. Leaving aside the patient, who is the centre of your concern, there are some very significant people with whom you are dealing.

Yourself and Isolation

Firstly, you must survive through this ordeal, otherwise the patient is at grave risk. Much of this book has been devoted to methods of your survival. Make sure that you read the chapter on "How Do the Relatives Cope."

Relatives and Friends

Realise that your relatives and friends want to help. They are also very frightened of what has occurred and will not know what to do. Also they will not want to intrude into what is often seen as a personal tragedy. They need to help, and you certainly need them. Therefore, bring them into the picture as early as possible and give them work to do. Start off slowly, arranging one to answer the phone, another to draw up the roster, another to co-ordinate the visiting, another to commence the diary. You will always have someone with whom you just like to talk. Cultivate all their talents, incorporate them into the work of the programme. Select one or two to arrange meetings every two or three weeks when you can all get together and discuss what is going on. There will always be some relatives who are negative. Do everything that you can to get them on-side. One person who is opposed can exert a powerful destructive influence.

I well recall the case of a young man whose mother was opposed to any therapy even though the rest of the family was positive. She really did prevent therapy from being given because of her antagonism. Sometimes, you have no alternative but to exclude the opposer, but do so in as sensitive a manner as possible. In fact, you will often find that there is no need to do anything as they will tend to drop out of active involvement without your intervention.

DO NOT ISOLATE YOURSELF FROM YOUR RELATIVES AND FRIENDS.

Relatives of Other Patients

It is very likely that you will become acquainted with the relatives of other patients. They can be a source of great comfort to you. They often share a common problem and understand what you are experiencing, and many long term and deep friendships are formed at this time of great stress. If they have a method of dealing with the strain of this time, allow them to share it with you and conversely, you should share with them.

Nursing Staff

Most nurses are great people. Do not get them off-side. They are caring and concerned and want to help. They too are finding their way in this world. They have good times and bad times. They want to do their work and be appreciated for it. They also have the "hands on" aspect of care. Their hands touch the patient more than anyone else's (except yours). You want them to be loving hands. You want the touch to be gentle. You want the care to be patient and kind. You must therefore treat them as you wish the patient to be treated. Show them that you appreciate their concern for the patient. Treat them with respect. Be patient with them. Try not to force them into a corner over their care of the patient. If you have difficulties then seek to resolve them rapidly. It is always a good idea to let the Charge Sister know when you are in the ward as a matter of courtesy and also because it establishes your presence. Treat the junior nurses with respect also. Word soon gets around the nursing staff as to how YOU deal with people.

The Social Worker

Select your Social Worker with care, for they can support you or can drain your energies. Seek to obtain one with some life experience and with whom you feel comfortable. Do not listen to those whom you feel are not on your wave length. If there is any attempt to split you or a family member off from the group, resist it. Ask for a change if necessary. The one you want is a person who will listen to you, even when you are unreasonable, and when you know that you are unreasonable, and will still not be critical of you, but will support you.

Physiotherapist and Occupational Therapists

These two disciplines have a great deal to offer the person who is brain-injured. If you can find exploratory therapists who will not stick rigidly to the party line, they can be of great benefit. They can help you with the programme and with its development. Be careful, however, of those who consider that there is only one right way to help the brain-injured. Mostly you will find that the hospital is so short of these therapists that they are only able to spend a limited time, often half an hour per day on any one patient. Do not try and force them to do more. If they can show you what to do with passive range of movement and give you any additional help, accept it, be grateful and realise that your own presence and hands are of the utmost benefit.

The Interpreter

If you are not fluent in the local language, your problems are multiplied greatly. In my dealings with the relatives of the brain injured, I am deeply concerned when dealing with someone who is a migrant. The system is difficult enough to deal with if you can speak the language, but almost impossible, if you do not. An interpreter becomes a valuable asset in such circumstances.

You must select an interpreter who is in harmony with you and your philosophy. You must ensure that he/she spends adequate time with you and is present at any meetings you have with the doctor or nursing staff. The interpreter should be bound by ethics which will mean that any information which s/he obtains is covered by professional secrecy. Your conversations will not therefore be voiced abroad.

If you have a friend who can interpret, this may even be better than using a hospital interpreter, since your friend may have more time. Do not however, use your friend if s/he is not proficient as an interpreter. S/he may still be of value, even so, just sitting in on any conversations and ensuring that you understand what is being said. This whole matter of language is far too serious to be dealt with inadequately.

THE MEDICAL PROFESSION

This is the power base of the whole health care system. The admission of patients, the investigation of patients, the diagnosis of patients, the treatment of patients and the transfer or discharge of patients is determined by this powerful group.

Because you will be treading into their area of competence with revolutionary ideas the whole process needs to be undertaken with tact and discretion and with a great deal of forethought and planning. The concept of the approach distance dealt with in Chapters 6 and 7 applies as much to the physician as it does to the patient. So move carefully. You are in "Tiger Country."

A. Identify the Physicians Involved

Firstly, you must identify who is the prime care controller of the patient. If the patient is in the Intensive Therapy Unit, it is likely to be the Director of that Unit especially if the injury has been a closed head injury and there has been either no need for surgery or only minor surgery. If there has been major cranial surgery, the controller of care is likely to be the neurosurgeon, certainly for the first few days after the surgery.

When the patient moves out of the Intensive Therapy Unit into a high dependency ward, the Intensive Care staff lose all control and the patient is the responsibility of the neurosurgeon who will maintain this authority for a period of weeks or months. In some cases there will be conflict between the physicians in Intensive Therapy and the neurosurgeon. Do not become caught in this.

B. Find out What Type of Person the Physician is

My advice to you is to obtain as much information about the attitudes of all care controllers as you can. This can frequently be picked up from the nursing staff, the social workers and relatives of other patients. You do not need to ask direct questions about their competence. In general, the standard of medical care in the neurosurgical and intensive care field is of the highest order. Often the answers will come to you if you ask what type of people they are.

C. Arrange a Meeting with the Physician

It is wise to meet the attending physicians separately. This is often difficult especially with the neurosurgeon, but it is worthwhile. Decide which person you feel most comfortable with and discuss the condition of the patient with him or her. Indicate that you wish to take an active part in the recovery of the patient and see what is the attitude to this proposal. Do not lay out an enormous proposal. Just see how the physician feels about it. If he or she is positive, then take it slowly, you do not need to give any more indications apart from your desire to be involved. If he/she wants more details, ask for time to put these in writing. This will allow time for all parties to consider what should be done.

D. How to Handle the Antagonistic Physician

If the physician is antagonistic, do not persevere with the matter at that time. Above all, maintain your cool. Do not let your "hot" brain jump out. If you find you are being blocked on a point, persevere only for a short time and then attempt to come from another direction. Appear to be reasonable at all times. Do all you can to prevent a confrontation. You are in a long struggle. You do not have to win every battle immediately. You are interested in winning the war.

If you are blocked seek out an alternative pathway. If necessary ask for a second opinion on the patient, meet with the other physician and see what the attitude is to the relative's involvement. If you feel it is the correct thing to do, have the patient transferred to the person who is most receptive to your approach.

Do this transfer early, before you have been labelled as a troublemaker by the profession. If you are labelled in this way, you may have difficulty obtaining another doctor willing to take over the care of the patient.

E. The Importance of Correct Preparation

In all your dealings with the profession, make sure that you are well prepared with all the knowledge you will need. Make sure that you are familiar with the Glasgow Coma Scale and where the patient is on it. Know what type of injury the patient has had. Know what drugs he or she is on and have it written down when they were commenced and what the dosage is. Do not go into an interview without having done your homework. Every time you see the physician, you are moving into his/her territory and you must be well prepared. The more you are prepared, the more you will be listened to.

F. The Use of a Mediator

It is often wise to take a friend, especially one skilled in negotiation. If confrontation appears inevitable you have three choices. One is to "cool it". Just hold off having any more contact with the physician for a couple of weeks. If you have time, this is often best. If you have not time to do this or the situation is serious, then you may need to have the services of a mediator. Seek out someone, especially in one of the other professions, Dentistry, Law, the Clergy, etc.to come with you and give you guidance. Your other alternative is to seek to have the patient transferred to another physician either in the same or another hospital.

MEDICAL ETHICS AND INFORMED CONSENT

The *Declaration of Geneva* of The World Medical Association binds the doctor with the words "The health of my patient will be my first consideration."

The question of Informed Consent is an important one in Medicine. Consent means that every diagnostic procedure or treatment given to the patient can only be given with the permission of the patient. Informed means that the information has been given to the patient in an accurate and understandable manner, including all the advantages, hazards and disadvantages of the diagnostic procedure or treatment.

There are many physicians who would agree that when Medicine has no more to offer, this fact should be made known to the relatives along with any alternatives, both proven and unproven.

Many physicians would see that the provision of a non-intrusive, apparently harmless attempt by the relatives and friends to arouse a patient from coma, is a reasonable thing to do.

The Helsinki Declaration of the World Medical Association (1975) II. Medical Research Combined with Professional Care (Clinical Research) states;

"The potential benefits, hazards and discomforts of a new method should be weighed against the advantages of the best current diagnostic and therapeutic techniques."

Since the results of the best current techniques are already known, these results should be made known to the relatives by the physician and the decision as to the action to be taken should remain with the relatives as legal guardian of the patient.

It may be possible for you to present to the physician the possibility that you would like him or her to be researching the whole process of coma arousal. The same section of the Helsinki Agreement states "In the treatment of the sick person, the doctor must be free to use a new diagnostic or therapeutic measure, if in his or her judgment it offers hope of saving life, re-establishing health or alleviating suffering."

THE LEGAL SYSTEM

The Law varies in each country. If you think that entering into medical territory is difficult, you will be confused even more by the legal profession. It is well worth seeking the best legal advice you can. This does not necessarily mean the most expensive. It means the most caring and competent. Seek this advice early. Maintain constant contact with your legal adviser. Do not assume that things are happening without knowing what is going on.

OTHER ORGANISATIONS

Other organisations can be of great help to you. They will provide a network of knowledge of how to deal with the problems which you have at present and also the difficulties which you will have to face in the future.

There is frequently more than one relevant organisation in each country and it is wise for you to check out the attitude and philosophy of each and what their aims are. Often you will hear derogatory remarks about some organisation. Store this information in your brain but do not be necessarily put off. This whole area is a very emotional one and there is a lot of "infighting", which is most unfortunate.

Often organisations will put out booklets which will help in deciding in which order you should approach them. Really you need to make a short list of the various organisations and work from it.

One other way to get preliminary information is to ask for the names of people who belong to the organisation and have been in a similar position to you. The organisation may be unwilling to give you names and phone numbers, but they may be prepared to get some one to telephone you. Of course, the best way is for you to make personal contact through friends with someone who has been in "your boat".

Having done all your preliminary checking, then go and look and see for yourself what the organisation has to offer. Do not make any quick decisions and always go and talk with some friends about what you have found.

The organisations which I am aware of are;

AUSTRALIA

1. The Australian Brain
   Foundation,
   7th Floor
   258 Little Bourke St.,
   Melbourne 3000.
   (03) 663-1591

2. Brain Injury Division
   4 Rutledge St.,
   Eastwood 2122
   (02) 85-1626

3. Headway Victoria
   763 High St.,
   East Kew.
   Melbourne 3102
   (03) 859-4977

4. The Australian Centre for
   Brain Injured Children
   52 Argyle St.
   St.Kilda.
   Melbourne. 3182
   (03) 534-8734

5. College for Development
   of Human Potential
   65 Badger Creek Road
   Healesville, 3777
   Australia
   (059) 623-084

THE UNITED KINGDOM

1. Headway Britain,
   200 Mansfield Rd.,
   Nottingham. NGI. 3HX.
   England
   (0602) 622-382

2. The British Life
   Assurance Trust (BLAT)
   BMA House, tavistock Square,
   London WC1H9JP
   01-3887976

THE UNITED STATES

1. The National Head
   Injury Foundation
   P.O. Box 567,
   Framingham, MA 01701
   U.S.A.
   (617) 879-7473.

2. Sandler-Brown Consultants
   612 Fitzwatertown Rd,
   Willow Grove,
   Pennsylvania, 19090,
   U.S.A.
   (215) 657-5250

3. The Institutes for the
   Achievement of Human
   Potential
   8801 Stenton Ave.,
   Philadelphia.
   Penna. 18118
   U.S.A.
   (215) 233-2050

4. New Medico Head Injury Systems
   113 Broad St.,
   Lynn. MA 01902
   1-800-343-1238

Conclusion

Like all systems, the health care system works best for those who know how to make the system work for them. This entails the gaining of knowledge on how the system works, clarifying of the problem to be engaged, the application of knowledge to the problem, the resistance of any attempt to be drawn into irrelevant fighting, the reduction of friction at every possible opportunity and the seeking not to make enemies.

Know what your objectives are at all times. Do your homework. There is much to be gained by victory. Defeat will mean unrelenting sorrow and anguish.

CONCLUSION

And if we truly value ourselves,
if we appraise the human difference
at its real worth,
how can we then
except in self defence or the defence of others
treat any other person or people as less than
precious.

Morton Hunt, *The Universe Within*, The Harvester Press, England. 1982

CONCLUSION

Introduction

"Less than precious?" Daily, throughout the world, many people are treated as less than precious. Organisations such as Amnesty International seek justice and freedom for people exist and strive to bring about the release of the captive. Condemnation of a person without trial or with a false trial is regarded as completely unthinkable and unacceptable in civilised countries.

And yet, many people who are severely brain injured are condemned to a lingering existence, often extending for years or even decades, because of the failure of our health care systems to look at the problem and to seek the solution.

How is this to be done? In the first instance, the very first instance, the present method of standing at arm's length (or at the foot of the bed), from the brain-injured person, must be changed.

Henri Nouwen, *The Wounded Healer* (Image Books, 1979), heads a chapter "Looking into the Fugitive's Eyes." He writes in a different context from this problem, but the message remains the same. He tells the story of a minister, who, torn between the survival of his village and the survival of one young man in wartime conditions, found guidance in the words," It is better that one man dies than that the whole people be lost." He proceeded to sacrifice the young man and when full of remorse was visited by an angel who asked, "What have you done?" He said, "I handed over the fugitive to the enemy." Then the angel said, "But don't you know that you handed over the Messiah?" "How could I know?" the minister replied anxiously. Then the angel said: "If, instead of reading your Bible, you had visited this young man just once, and looked into his eyes, you would have known."

We, too, are challenged to look into the eyes of the young men and women of today who are brain-injured, whom we make into the outcasts and fugitives of our civilization and health care systems.

The Caring Professions and the Patient

I have emphasized in previous chapters, the importance of eye contact as a significant indicator that the channel of communication is open between people. I have stressed the idea that this applies equally to the brain-injured and the non-brain injured. Because we, in the caring professions, are the powerful ones and the patient is the powerless one, it is our right and responsibility and privilege to be the seekers, the initiators of this communication. It is no longer right for us to look from afar off in a cursory fashion at the patient who is in prolonged coma. We need to come close, to touch, to feel, to see, to bind ourselves to the patient who is in

265

such a terrible predicament. We need to look into the eyes. If we see nothing the first time or the third time or the tenth time, this should not dissuade us from looking. And when we look, we should aim to see. We should not look with a closed mind.

The plea by Professor J. Moore, *Recovery of Function: Theoretical Considerations for Brain Injury Rehabilitation*, Ed. Paul Bach-y-Rita,(Hans Huber, Publishers, Bern, Stuttgart, Vienna, 1980) is relevant. She writes, "Do we need thousands of written case histories . . . . . . before we are willing to open up the intellectual barriers of our minds and begin to listen?

"Are thousands of case histories necessary before we are willing to accept and recognise the fascinating potentials that are available within the nervous system for stimulating and enhancing the recovery process through multiple therapeutic techniques, each geared to individual patients needs?

"Certainly the hundreds if not thousands, of research articles concerning the effects of sensory deprivation and enriched environments . . . . . . should constitute a reliable basis upon which we can reject the outdated and time worn classical concepts concerning the structure and function of the nervous system and readily accept new ideas."

The strength of opinion held by Dr A.Bricolo, Dr S.Turazzi and Dr G.Feriotti from Verona is one with which I totally agree. In the *Journal of Neurosurgery* (Prolonged Post Traumatic Coma, 1980: 52;625-634) they write; "It makes it mandatory to continue rehabilitation relentlessly in all cases", and "What makes the final balance sheet so dismaying is . . . the high incidence of outcomes implying severe disablement and making the survivors totally dependent on others and capable of suffering and causing grief."

They also write, "We are prepared to admit that this may be due also, or even, prevalently to the inadequacy of rehabilitation therapy."

They end their paper with the following, "Thus, in our opinion, the problem is not so much the cost of treatment, as improving our ability to avoid secondary cerebral lesions in the early course of as many patients as possible, and to create the conditions for maximum recuperation of nervous function and social rehabilitation."

Point by point, what they are saying is;
1. It is essential to continue rehabilitation in all cases.
2. It is dismaying to have such a high incidence of disabled people.
3. This high incidence may be due to the inadequacy of our rehabilitation services.
4. One approach to the problem is to reduce the second insult to the brain (i.e., restoring internal environment).
5. The other approach is to provide the optimum conditions to restore brain function and social rehabilitation (i.e., restoring external environment).

The articles by these authors are nearly a decade old, and it is obvious that a ferment of change within the professions has commenced.

The *New York Times* is aware of some of the problems which stem from traditional lack of care accorded the brain-injured and also aware of the new thought which is slowly eroding away fixed thinking. In its supplement to the edition of 27th June 1982, it says; "There are professionals today who take a dramatically different view. They maintain that even the most primitive sign of sentience may offer the opportunity for rehabilitation.

"A leading supporter of that proposition is Dr Sheldon Berrol, Assistant Clinical Professor of Rehabilitation at the University of California, and Chairman of a national medical task force on head injury. Dr Berrol is exploring the potential of a damaged brain's undamaged parts to adopt new functions."

Dr Nathan Cope, Director of the Head Injury Unit, santa Clara Medical Centre, San Jose, California, acknowledges "If you put the patient in an environment that promotes change and look two years later, you'll see change. Forty seven percent of the people in the programme, who by normal standards would be judged as reaching their limit continue to improve."

The Caring Professions and the Relatives

We must also look into the eyes of relatives of the brain injured with feeling and compassion. It is not enough for the most junior doctor to be the source of information about the patient. The relatives need the care of the person who is really in charge. They do not want to be fobbed off into the bottom of the medical hierarchy. Their world has been shattered, they are afloat on a sea of disaster, buffeted by the unknown, often isolated from their support groups, bereft of guidance, without any knowledge of the termination of their journey. It is no wonder that they demonstrate stressful behaviour.

What they need has been briefly and eloquently expressed in John Haggai's book *My Son Johnny* (Tyndale House Publishers, Illinois, 1978) with the words, "How important it is, to reach out in love and encouragement, to someone whose life has gone into a place of darkness."

They need information given to them in an understandable and deliberate and compassionate way.

To the Relatives and Friends

Very recently, I had a beautiful girl brought to me as a patient. The family was in chaos. The girl had been injured some eighteen months before, had been admitted to a local hospital with a severe brain injury and transferred to a major city teaching hospital where she had been expertly treated for her life-threatened state. At a suitable time she had been transferred to the rehabilitation section of a hospital in her own city, transferred from there to another hospital for further treatment, and sent back to the city into a specialist rehabilitation hospital. From there she had been sent to another institution of the same type where she had remained for some months. The mother, father and brother along with the patient had finally arrived on my doorstep, having been told that nothing more could be done and that they must find a nursing home in which to place their daughter. The girl was in good health and appeared to understand everything that was being said. I checked her over. She was certainly out of coma and gave every indication of awareness. She attempted to answer questions and even though she had great difficulty, she was able to communicate.

With the patient and all members of the family in the room along with a senior nurse, I began the discussion as to what should be done. The first question was to the girl enquiring as to whether she wished to go into a nursing home for the rest of her life. She, quite rightly, said no. I then went through the story of the occurrences since the accident, pointing out to all how the health care systems undertaking retrieval and survival had worked effectively. I then pointed out how ineffective had been the attempt to solve the problems of restoring the functions that the patient required to undertake independent living. I stressed that the health care system had failed them repeatedly. The patient had been in four hospitals supposedly in an attempt to rehabilitate her and had failed to do so. The last hospital had "washed their hands" of her. The health care system, having attempted to solve the problem and failed wished to dispose of the patient by shifting her out of the system into the discard area of a nursing home.

I put it to the parents. The system had failed. There was no chance that the system would succeed. It had made four attempts and still wished to discard their daughter. I pointed out that perhaps it was time to take matters into their own hands. Was there any logic in doing anything else? They understood what I said, resolved to take the initiative, bring their daughter home, seek the support of their townspeople and set up a programme in their own home. As of this moment the girl is doing well.

All of the above sounds terribly critical of the system. It is not meant to be. What I want to emphasise is that patients surviving with severe brain injury are relatively new on the medical scene. The system is not yet aware enough of the problems of these patients let alone geared up to deal with them.

It will take years for the change in attitude and gaining of knowledge to be strong enough to bring about change. It might never change. The prolonged care of the brain-injured must compete financially with all other health requirements. It is unlikely that the prolonged input of capital and personnel resources needed for the restoring of function can compete against the newsmaking drama of heart transplants or cancer cures, etc.

In any case, YOU cannot wait. I have constantly stressed through this book the importance of the relative. YOU are the one who views the patient as the most precious. YOU are the one with the close bond to the patient. YOU are the one who has the maximum incentive to get the patient better. YOU are the one who has the time commitment. Do not rely on anyone else. Go for it yourself, always seeking harmony with those of the health care professions who will listen to you. Do not spend time on the others.

Does this Book Fit Within a Scientific Framework and Why was it Written?

It was the Nobel Prize winner, Sir Peter Medawar who wrote: "Scientific reasoning is a constant interplay or interaction between hypotheses and the logical explanations they give rise to; a restless to-and-fro motion of thought, the formulation and reformulation of hypotheses, until we arrive at a hypothesis which, to the best of our prevailing knowledge, will satisfactorily meet the case.

"Scientific reasoning is a kind of dialogue between the possible and the actual, between what might be and what is in fact the case." Medawar, P. *The Art of the Soluble* (London:Methuen and Co., 1967).

Dr H. Judson, in *In Search for Solutions*(Hutchinson and Co, London, 1980) writes "Passion is indispensable for creation, no less in the sciences than in the arts. Medawar once described it in a talk addressed to young scientists. You must feel in yourself an exploratory impulsion — an acute discomfort at incomprehension. This is the rage to know."

I have raged to know since 1979. The answers to my questions were inadequate or insulting as I sought to know what was to be done about brain injury.

I started to see the brain-injured as people caught in the ultimate dungeon by the disaster which had befallen them. I touched them and looked into their eyes and anguished over their plight. I sought to bring them to the attention of my colleagues.

The relatives are the key to the diagnosis and the treatment. From the relatives, I learnt to look with eyes that see. Whenever I speak to a relative I am searching for what they know, often intuitively. I have used their eyes, their hands, their brain to guide me in this search. I have also learnt the strength that is within all; the courage, the endurance, the patience, the faith, the hope, and the love which is the essence of existence.

The Moral Problems

There are many moral problems associated with this work. In the first instance, there is the problem in the intensive care ward — whether to save the life of a person who may become vegetative or severely disabled. This is an enormously difficult decision since the measuring devices are not absolute.

Second, is the fact that the relatives should have the right to intervene with the patient and should be provided with the tools to attempt coma arousal if they so wish and if it does not appear to be having any harmful effect on the patient.

Third, is the problem of what to do with the patient who is still in coma after two weeks and likely to go into prolonged coma. Who should make the decisions? In Chapter 23, I have spoken about the importance of the relative's involvement in this decision making and the fact that they should be provided with all information concerning the orthodox method of treating the patient and any alternatives. I have stressed that the relatives should be allowed to make an Informed Consent. To deny them this right, I consider is intolerable, immoral and unethical and not in keeping with the spirit of the Helsinki Agreement of The World Medical Association.

Fourth, is the lack of therapy given in many rehabilitation hospitals. Many physicians, nursing staff and paramedical staff would dearly love to increase the amount of therapy given to the patients but are denied resources. In the final analysis, it is the politicians of the country who bear responsibility for this enormous lack. Their attention must be brought to their responsibilities in this matter.

Finally, what of the patient who does stay severely brain-injured and totally dependent? For them, adequate, loving, caring help should be available within hospices of high nursing standard. These should provide relatives' support groups to help cope with the unrelenting bereavement which is the lot of these unfortunate people.

Is this Book Complete?

The answer, of course, is No! It is a beginning only — a first step into the "Medical Desert" of brain injury. Undoubtedly, as many of my friends say, "It is like blunderbuss therapy." The medical future will see the establishment of proper inputs, measured accurately and recorded. It will see the defining of the initial point of awareness and will accurately map the arousal from coma and the correct endpoint of coma. It will measure the pre trauma personality of the patient against recovery. It will measure the input of the relatives, the effect of love and care. It will measure aspects of the environment which today we do not even recognize as significant and most importantly it will see the patient as a person who has an "approach distance" which must be protected at all times and which must not be abused.

At this stage, much of what is discussed is still theory waiting to be put into practice and weighed and measured. The words of Dr Judson apply, "A theory, like a map, must fit together data that are inevitably incomplete, always at some level approximate, sure to contain mistakes. At the same time, the map connects up the information in many directions."

Leaving aside the sexist language, the beauty of Whittier's hymn guides us all.

O brother man, fold to thy heart thy brother:
where pity dwells, the peace of God is there;
to worship rightly is to love each other,   John Greenleaf Whittier
each smile a hymn, each kindly deed a prayer.   1807-1892

INDEX

271